I SURVIVED

From Cancer to the Runway

A Unique Survival Story

Erica Campbell

Written/Published by Campbell, Erica (www.ericasurvived.com)

Edited by Ashleigh Wilkerson

Author front cover photo by LeRoy Armstead

Author back cover photo by Drew Xeron

Formatting and cover design by Maria Ann Green

ISBN: 978-0-578-78082-5

LCCN Library of Congress Control Number: 2020921000

This book is dedicated to:

My Mom and Dad who has loved me my entire life. For all their support throughout my entire cancer survival journey. To my siblings for their continuous love and support. To my amazing oncology doctor and her entire team for being there every step of the way to see me to the finish line. To my Beautiful Cancer Warriors. Most importantly and never least, my Lord and Savior, Jesus Christ for hearing my cries and saving my life.

Thank You.

Table of Contents

Introduction

Cancer. Anxiety. Depression. Beauty. They all connect with me in a unique and very scary way.

I never believed in a million years that I'd go through something so challenging. Why me? That's something I've thought about on various occasions. How did this happen to me? How was I the lucky number picked out of so many? Was there something that I did wrong? Where did this come from? What happens now? Should I have changed something in my diet? What are the chances that it had to be me? Don't get me wrong, I've been through my share of experiences just as the next person, but this is totally different. This is a level I never planned on reaching.

This is something you're not really taught about. Aware yes, but you don't think about the possibilities of it happening to you. It's a very unpleasant surprise; a total disaster if you will.

I just kept trying to remember that everything happens for a reason, and sometimes the reason doesn't make any sense. I just kept thinking "Why me? WHY ME?!" I know that no one is perfect, and most of the things we are faced with are needed to get to our final destination. So what did I do? Well, I'd say my approach was similar to being a boxer. That's right, I got in the ring and I gave it my all. I didn't stop. For every obstacle that came my way, I met it head on. Did I cry from time to time? Of course I did. I can't tell you how many tears I wiped down and across my face. But I had courage and the heart to wipe them away because I wanted a second chance. I wanted to take back control of my life and my body. That's right, I said my life and my body. I had to remind myself that both belong to me and I can do anything I put my mind to. I can get through anything. I wanted to show not only myself but anyone dealing with even a fourth of what I'm about to share with you, that the impossible is beyond possible. You can get through it. How is that so? That's what you're probably wondering right? Well us being here together right now means I did it. I survived! I didn't back down and I didn't stop until I beat CANCER!

I need you to understand that something that was sent to break me, actually is the very thing continuing to make me. It's continuing to make me stronger. You see, I now know life and the meaning of health in a totally different light. When I talk about being blessed, I count this victory more than twice. I look in the mirror every day and I see a winner. I see a winner because I didn't give up and God's plan on my life is far greater than I have ever imagined. But I won't forget. I won't ever go a day without being thankful for where I am now. I suffered through more than most can handle. At this very moment I can still remember everything. I take pride and joy in that.

None of my tears were in vain. I didn't allow it. I want too much out of life. I always did. I am a fighter. I am determined. I remember the mornings, the afternoons, and every appointment. I remember the sun shining bright even when my days felt so dark.

* * *

*I*t was spring. The grass was cut low and there were blooming flowers everywhere. There was always a cool breeze. I can still feel it right across my toes. Cute sandals were my favorite comfort shoes. I remember wearing my favorite pair of jeans. I always had on a loose shirt. The breeze ran through it as well. My hair now cut low with pretty curls bringing out my round face. I can smell the hospital. I can taste the food too. I can see my eyes still tired but hopeful. I hear every single word bouncing off the walls. I hear their voices. All of my doctors spoke so patiently with me. I still feel their concern for my well-being. I feel my gown covering my body too. I see my jeans and my top folded and placed by the counter. My legs still dangle. My hands still fold and sit nicely on my lap. I can see so many people who look just like me. I still feel their pain. Although there for different reasons, we all wanted a positive take away. I still pray for them, and I thank God that I got mine. Being told that I'm cancer free will always be the greatest memory by far.

I have many days where I battle with depression and anxiety attacks which stemmed from my fight against cancer. To add to that, I also battle with my own set of beauty insecurities because of the changes in my features such as facial hyperpigmentation (skin discoloration). I often worry about how others may view me if I went without makeup. I wonder if they would look at me and think I'm weird or even worst, think that I was ugly. It's tough being a girly girl because we as women want to be beautiful and feel attractive in every way. As little girls, we want to be princesses. As women we want to be queens. Although our looks don't define either of these things, this is what we are taught growing up. This is what we encounter every day in society, and it makes most of us feel that this is the way we should be. We put our kid-friendly makeup on our little faces as little girls. Similar to this notion as women, we apply all types of products to cover blemishes that come with life changes (aging, CANCER, family traits, etc.) hoping to look beautiful for our own personal reasons. These tough challenges are derived from transformative circumstances. Most of us share some of the same adversities. Sometimes it's unexpected and sometimes coping with the unexpected can be difficult. The world can make you feel as if you're crazy or insane for having these life-altering situations.

Now let's get to the real stuff: how cancer sent me on the rollercoaster ride of my life. Let me take you to the beginning where my life changed forever.

Names of doctors, nurses, and others have been changed to protect identity.

Part 1

Chapter 1:
The Beginning

*I*t all started in November 2012. I began coughing persistently for days. I took several over the counter meds like cough syrups and Halls but nothing seemed to help this ongoing, irritating cough. I did everything in order to keep myself from stressing. As we all know in many cases stress alone can only add fuel to the fire. Besides, we all get a cold from time to time right? After about a week and lots of effort, I decided to make an appointment with my primary physician to see what was going on. I didn't want to assume, but I also didn't want to take any chances with my health. The annoying cough seemed to be lingering and I've always known it's much better to be safe than sorry. My doctor's office scheduled my appointment for the following day and I couldn't wait. I was ready for an answer. I knew that my doctor would at least prescribe something better than what I was currently taking at home. That alone could have been a big factor in whatever difficulties I was experiencing. Either way, I was anxious to say the least. I arrived at the office that next afternoon. I checked in with the front desk receptionist, and waited in the lobby until I was called back to see my physician. Moments later Nurse Rachelle called out to me. She escorted me to one of the empty exam rooms. She took my vitals and asked me why I was there. I explained to her about my ongoing cough. She was very attentive. While I spoke she typed notes into the computer system. Once she finished she informed me that Dr. Smith would be in shortly.

Here I am sitting in the exam room waiting on my doctor and thinking to myself, "I hope that he can prescribe something to knock this right out." Dr. Smith came into the exam room. We talked a bit about my symptoms. He said that I have a dry cough. He prescribed Robitussin and antibiotics. He said that I should take them for several days. "Short and sweet appointment" I thought to myself. I left after Dr. Smith gave me my written prescription slip. Then I went to the CVS pharmacy near my house to get my medication. I was eager to get this cough and possible infection under control. I stayed on the meds like clockwork. I was taking one antibiotic pill per day and cough syrup every 4 hours. But somehow it wasn't working. The cough wouldn't budge. It started to take a lot out of me. My energy was beginning to drain from my body. There was so much strain that I began to feel sluggish. Over the last few weeks or so, my colleagues and friends noticed that I was losing weight. I thought nothing of it and took it as the grace of God that I was able to do so without working out. (I know, isn't that a laugh out loud moment? LOL) Anyway, as I began to go deeper into what could be causing such an annoying cough, I realized I was also going through night sweats. I was slowing down. Preparing for work in the mornings became much harder than usual. Even simple tasks such as standing in the shower, felt strenuous. But again, I blamed it on what I believed to be a cold. I figured it was turning into the flu.

A week went by and I have taken all of the medications prescribed by Dr. Smith. I still wasn't in the clear. I was coughing every few seconds and feeling very ill at this point. I decided to make another appointment with him to get further observation. A few days passed and it was time for us to meet again. This time he suggested that I have a Computerized Axial Tomography (CAT) scan (also known as a CT scan) performed. I trusted him, and I was very proactive. I immediately called the radiology center that he referred. I made an appointment set for that coming Friday. Of course I had lots of things going through my mind at the time. I wasn't sure how to feel just yet. I went from having a cold to needing a scan, but either way I was a step further to getting my answer.

It was Friday afternoon and I just left work for the day. I was headed to my CAT scan appointment. I was so nervous thinking about the unknown. But I didn't let it stop me. I had to remain level headed. I prepared for the unthinkable, but hoped for the best. I arrived at the radiology center. I signed in and waited to have my name called by one of the technicians. As I was waiting, I was wondering to myself, "What could possibly be wrong with me?"

After a few minutes, my name was called by one of the techs to come to the back. The technician explained the CAT scan procedure to me. She asked me to get undressed from the waist up. Then she walked me into the room where the big weird CAT scan machine was. I laid on the cold hard table. She asked me to put my arms above my head. Just a little while later, the table moved into the round tube right behind my head. I am not a fan of being in closed spaces. Those five minutes felt more like a lifetime. The tech proceeded to bring the table back out from the tube. When I began to get up, I felt really stiff. The examiner came into the room where I was and explained that the results would be sent over to my doctor's office for review. She said within a few days I should receive a response. I thanked her and began to put my clothes back on and then I left.

Before I had the chance to make it home, my phone rang. It was Dr. Smith! He stated that my CAT scan showed some signs of Pneumonia. He said that I needed to schedule another test with a contrast to get a better look at the prognosis. I was relieved at how quickly I was given my response, but I wasn't happy about the results at all. I didn't want to go through that same procedure all over again. "But what was I to do?" I thought to myself. I had to know if I had pneumonia or maybe something else was going on. So I decided to do as told. At the conclusion of our conversation, I called and made another appointment for the following week. At this point, I was very scared. I knew the only thing I could do was wait and see what happens next.

It was the day for my second CAT scan. Just like before, I signed in and waited to be called. After having another uncomfortable scan like the previous, I was hoping that the results came back differently this time. I left the radiology center. Dr. Smith called with the results but this time he stated something totally different from the last results. He said that my scans show enlarged lymph nodes surrounding my lungs which may be the primary reason for my ongoing cough. I asked Dr. Smith what exactly does that mean, and what can be done to treat the issue? He asked me to come back to his office to speak further. He said there was more to it than just taking some prescribed medicine. So here I was in my car driving home, taking in every detail that he just explained and wondering to myself, "What was really going on with me?"

My ride felt very long and I couldn't even remember how I got from one part of town to my driveway. I had to admit to myself that I was beyond perturbed. As the days went by tension slid all throughout my body. I couldn't help it. I tried my hardest to remain optimistic, but I was distressed. I guess I worried myself to death wondering why I needed to talk in person. I worried even more when learning about lymph nodes. I shared this small piece of information with those close to me. They tried their hardest to ease my anxiety. They told me it would be okay and not to worry myself. But of course, that part was hard. I wouldn't be able to relax until I knew for sure what I was dealing with on the inside. Not to mention on top of all of this news, I was still coughing uncontrollably. I was still very sluggish and unable to fully feel like myself. As the days went on, the pain remained. It was a struggle to get ready for work each morning. I refused to be defeated. Although it took much longer than I was used to, I still pushed myself in order to carry out my daily routine. Sometimes it felt like I couldn't breathe. I found myself experiencing shortness of breath regularly. Anytime I would walk up my stairs at home or even a short distance, I would feel myself out of breath as if I ran miles. I wasn't quite understanding what was happening to my body, but I knew I would find out when I met with Dr. Smith again.

The day was here for him and I to sit down. Just like the previous weeks, I was uneasy. I was sitting in the exam room waiting for him to come talk to me. I couldn't help but to wonder what he was going to say. I wondered if he had new information about my CAT scan prognosis. When he finally came in the room, he explained that my results led him to believe that I either had Sarcoidosis or Lymphoma. To be certain, I would need to see a specialist for further observation. I've heard about Sarcoidosis because of the comedian Bernie Mac. I remember he mentioned that he had it. However, I didn't know a lot about the disease. I had no clue what it really was until Dr. Smith said two of the scariest words of my life, "Lymphoma Disease". I looked at him in disbelief for a few seconds before asking how he came up with both possibilities. He explained that because of my test results and with research, my body showed symptoms for both diseases. He referred me to a specialist that I should take my results to. He said this would help to see if a biopsy should be performed to exclude one or the other. He said it would benefit me to the point that it could possibly exclude both. I was given a referral to see a specialist through John Hopkins Medical and then I left my doctor's office. I was really down about what was just explained to me. "Sarcoidosis!" "Cancer!" "Not me, NOT ME!"

For the rest of the day, I researched both diseases on google. I worried and stressed until I forced myself to go to sleep early that evening. The next morning as soon as the specialist office opened, I called to make an appointment. My consultation was scheduled for the following week. The more time I had, the more my thoughts consumed me. I was scared about the outcome. I was distraught trying to go over the possibilities. I knew I would suffer until I was able to see the specialist to go over my results a little more in detail. In the beginning when I did, I still wasn't too sure how much it helped. I was confused by everything that I was told. To think that it may be a chance I could be sick with cancer and if so, what was going to be my chances of survival? All I knew about cancer was that most people died from it, and only some survived. Even crazier, my Auntie was just diagnosed with Lymphoma a few shorts months ago. That was my only encounter with this type of cancer. So of course, because it was someone else going through it, I didn't know much about the disease. Now that it could be me, I was a bit more concerned.

Days and days of worry went by. Although it seemed like it took so long, it was finally the day for my appointment with the specialist. I would get to see what my fate would be. I checked in at the front desk and was asked by the receptionist to have a seat until my name was called. If this didn't seem like a bad case of déjà vu. It was always the same steps before seeing the doctors. Not long after sitting, I was called back into an exam room by the assistant nurse. She took my vitals and told me that Dr. Willington would be in shortly and then she left the room. A couple minutes later Dr. Willington came in to see me. He wanted to discuss my CAT scan results from the previous weeks. He stated that he took a look at my results before I arrived and noticed that there were enlarged lymph nodes around my lungs.

He said that due to his observation and my ongoing cough he thought that it would be best to have a surgical biopsy. This would further explain why the lymph nodes were enlarged. This would also explain why the cough hadn't disappeared as well.

I was at Dr. Willington's office for an hour discussing how the surgery would be performed. Now to pick the time and day. We chose December 3rd, 2012. It's just a few weeks away. I wasn't so happy about it. I wasn't so happy about any of it to be honest. I gathered myself and left his office an emotional wreck. I couldn't fully comprehend what just happened during our conversation and what was about to happen in a few weeks when my biopsy surgery is performed. As I sat in my car for a few moments, all I could think was, "Now this is beginning to be more serious than I thought?" I had no choice but to get my family involved so I called my Mom and broke the news to her first. She was in shock as she began to ask all types of questions. Then she stated that she hopes that everything was ok. So did I. My body was telling me something totally different from what I was thinking. It was hard not to be scared and assume the worst. I had never had surgery before besides having a bunion removed years ago. So this was something very different that I was about to experience for the first time in my life.

The symptoms for Lymphoma stuck out more to me. I was physically experiencing them all. I was enduring the unexplained night sweats, loss of weight, fatigue, persistent coughing and the overall ill health feeling. In the back of my mind I was thinking, "This may be Lymphoma and if so, then what?" As the weeks went by in a blink of an eye, it was the day I could be told I was seriously ill and sick with Cancer.

Chapter 2:
Things Didn't Go Too Well

*I*t was December 3rd, 2012, the day of my biopsy surgery. It was early in the morning. Both my Mom and Dad drove me to the hospital where I would have my surgery performed. I was a nervous wreck the entire ride. We were headed to Howard County Hospital. Once we arrived, I went to check in. I wasn't prepared for what happened next. I was told that I have a $500 insurance deductible to pay before surgery. I've had health insurance for some time now. I've never had to use my coverage outside of my annual doctors' appointments or minor issues. I've never faced any real medical needs where a deductible was involved. I knew little about medical coverage to be quite honest. I asked the receptionist if there was something that could be done so that I could have the surgery. I did not have $500 to give at this time and it was urgent that I got this biopsy surgery done. I needed to know if I was sick with cancer or not.

The receptionist asked me to take a seat for a moment while she spoke with the financial department. Some time went by and someone came to get me. I was going to speak to someone about my payment options before surgery. I explained to the individual in the financial department that I didn't have that kind of money at that time and needed a payment option. After going over my choices, I was able to finance my biopsy surgery with a monthly payment plan. After all of my paperwork was completed, I went back to the lobby where my parents were waiting and told them what happened. After a few moments in the lobby, I was called back to prep for my surgery which at this point was running a little behind because of the insurance issue.

I'm sitting in a room with my hospital gown on and with this IV in my right arm. I'm waiting for someone from the surgery staff to take me into the surgical room. At this point, I am really nervous and terrified. Before I was taken down to surgery, I was administered a special drug to suppress my persistent cough. It was to prevent me from choking while undergoing surgery. I was thinking to myself, "I wish I could have had that same drug all this time dealing with this crazy cough." Shortly after, I was taken back by a couple assistants to the surgery room. As I lay there undergoing numerous tasks, I was staring off at the ceiling silently praying to myself. I kept praying until the anesthesia kicked in.

"Ms. Campbell," a voice kept calling out to me. I was sleep for hours. I was still pretty out of it too. I was looking up at the lights over my head. I felt like I was in an episode of the Twilight Zone. Two of the technicians transferred me to a recovering room. I sat for about 30 minutes or so before Dr. Willington would come in to talk to me about my results. Time went by and the recovery nurse checked on me a few times. Dr. Willington soon followed. He had unpleasant news. My surgery was unsuccessful. I was looking in disbelief as I couldn't understand why or how this could be. I asked him how that could be possible? He explained because of the type of procedure that was performed, there wasn't enough of the lymph node removed. This prevented a guarantee of a successful biopsy. I said to him, "Well, there's something going on with me so now what?" Dr. Willington said that I would have to get another biopsy performed by another surgical doctor. This one would be a little more intense. A small incision would be cut across my neck to take a larger lymph node. "What in the world," is what my face expression was saying as I was listening to Dr. Willington explain everything to me.

Dr. Willington referred me to an expert at St. Agnes Hospital in Baltimore, MD. After that he walked away. I sat there mentally, physically, and emotionally in pain. I didn't understand why I had to go through such grief just to find out if I had cancer. It felt like a never-ending maze. I just wanted a clear answer so that I could move forward with the next steps. I still wouldn't allow myself to be crushed. I admit it was overwhelming, but I wasn't defeated. The recovery nurse came back to check on me once again. She asked a few questions to make sure I wasn't dizzy. She wanted to make sure that I was well enough to get dressed before I was discharged. I assured the nurse that I was fine. She helped me get dressed so that I could meet my parents in the lobby. Once I was reunited with my Mother and Father, I told them what I was told by Dr. Willington. They didn't understand how my surgery wasn't successful. They just said "Okay" and did everything in their power to support me during this unimaginable journey.

My parents drove home. Soon as I got in the door I immediately made a call to the new consultant's office. It was time for the hot seat yet again to obtain details for my second procedure. The secretary gave me a date that same week. I couldn't believe I was going through all of this back and forth with so many visits and surgeries. After a few days, I went to St. Agnes Hospital for my consultation with Dr. Henderson, the new surgical doctor. I walked up to the front desk to get a visitors sticker and continued to Dr. Henderson's office.

It seemed like the longest walk ever. Or maybe that was just my nerves. I became so familiar with this difficult routine, yet each time worry still managed to travel with me. While still walking, I managed to block out the fear of not knowing what to expect for the moment. Finally I made it! I had to check in at yet another front desk of course. After that I sat in the waiting area. Just like the times before I was frightened. I heard my name called which meant it was my turn again. I got up and walked over to the nurse. We made our way down the hall to the room. Dr. Henderson greeted me with a firm hand shake. Then he directed me to have a seat across from his bureau. We began to discuss everything that has transpired since my first appointment back in November up until now. He was prepared. Before I arrived he went over my CAT scan and my biopsy results. Then he went into a deeper discussion about his role, the procedure he was going to perform, and overall what to expect. We also talked about a surgery date and time within a few weeks. I was confident in his abilities. The conversation was very informative. Although still quite nervous, I left his office thinking to myself, "I hope that nothing else goes wrong moving forward and that this surgery is successful."

I began receiving calls from my insurance provider about some coverage issues. After a few stressful conversations with them, I canceled my insurance coverage all together. With that happening, I had to also cancel my upcoming surgery date with Dr. Henderson. I had to wait until I was able to get new coverage in the New Year. This was all becoming very overwhelming. On top of everything else that I was trying to wrap my head around, I was still feeling really sick, and coughing non-stop.

Some days were easier than others. Some days I felt more pain. Other days I coughed more than usual. Somehow despite every obstacle I kept going. I knew I had no other choice. The bumps in the road in regards to finances, appointments, and everything else in between couldn't stop me. I refused to give up so easily. I refused to give up at ALL.

Just as before, the days and time continued to fly and here I was walking into the New Year. I can't believe January was already here. The great news is that I had new health insurance coverage to get things back in order. I still needed to have my biopsy surgery. I was ready to call Dr. Henderson's office to request a new date. Unfortunately the secretary said that Dr. Henderson was booked with surgeries. The next available date was on March 28th, 2013.- WOW!! I had no other choice so I went with the available date. There really wasn't too much that I could do to change things. The next few months went by in what seemed to be the slowest time ever. My days seemed longer. I felt like I was counting the hours, the minutes, even the seconds. It also didn't help that the stress of my sickness became worse. I felt like my health was quickly declining. That made me think that "Maybe I do have cancer…" but I wouldn't know for sure until March.

Chapter 3:

The Moment My Life Changed...Forever

*I*t was finally March and I was thrilled and nervous at the same time. I was getting closer to my surgery date. It was the end of my work week. For months I've been dealing with a lot. One of my good girlfriends asked me if I wanted to go out for some food and cocktails. I didn't want to drink. One of my other complications was having lower back pains when I consumed any alcohol. I also wasn't having much of an appetite these days., but I reluctantly agreed . I wanted to get out so I could take my mind off of what was currently going on in my life. My girlfriend set the place and time. I told her that I would be there. When I got home from work that afternoon, I wasn't feeling 100% well. I was feeling sick to my stomach. I barely wanted to move. I was so dizzy. I told myself that I would push through anyway to enjoy a night out with friends.

I showered and got dressed to head out for the evening. As I was leaving my housing community, I vomited all over myself. I started to feel severely hot and very nauseous. I was sitting in the middle of the road crying and panicking. I called my girlfriend to tell her what was happening, and that I wasn't going to make it. She understood and told me to get back home to rest. After we hung up, I called my Mom to see if she and my Dad could take me to the hospital. She replied that he wasn't home and to call him to see where he was because he had the car. I then tried calling my Dad but he wasn't near. I called another girlfriend that lived nearby to see if she was home to take me to the hospital. She said she was about to pull into her apartment complex and that she would take me to the emergency room. I told her that I needed to change my clothes first and then I would head over to her house shortly. I drove back up to my house so that I could change. As I was trying to get into my home, my key broke off in the front door lock. I broke down into tears right there at my front door. I took a few moments to pull myself together before getting back into my car and driving to my girlfriend's place. My clothes were covered in vomit. When I arrived, I called her to come out but by this time I started to feel somewhat better. I headed to her door to go in for a few. At this point I can't get into my house. I'll have to wait for my Dad to take off the lock with the broken key in it.

Although I felt ok, my girlfriend insisted that I needed to get checked out. So much had occurred over the last few months. I agreed and she then took me to Southern MD Hospital. It was just 15 minutes down the beltway. We arrived at the hospital and I checked into the E.R. with the front desk. They told me to have a seat until I was called back. About 20 minutes went by and an associate called me back to have my vitals checked. Then I was sent back out to the waiting area. I was told I would be called back for further observation shortly after. It was after 10pm by this time. While I waited, I called my parents to let them know that I was at the hospital. They were headed up to meet me there. I was finally called to the back again by an E.R Nurse. She escorted me to a bed with a privacy curtain and advised me to change into a hospital gown. As I laid there in a hospital bed waiting for a doctor to come see me, I just couldn't help to feel jittery. A few moments went by before an E.R. doctor came in to talk to me about what I was experiencing. I explained what happened leading up to this day and that I am scheduled to have a biopsy surgery the following week. With that being said, the E.R. doctor stated that he wanted to have a CAT scan of his own done. He wanted to see if anything has changed to cause these sudden events that occurred a few hours ago.

I was taken back to the CAT scan room by a technician. Shortly after my scan, I returned to the hospital bed where I was earlier. My Mom was brought back to see what was going on with me. Not long after she came in, the E.R. doctor came back to explain my CAT scan results. He stated that although I was not officially diagnosed yet, it did in fact look like I have cancer.

The CAT scan showed that the cancer has spread throughout my entire upper body. In that quick moment, I felt my body go numb as he was saying the word "Cancer" out loud to me. He asked if I was still working. I told him yes. He advised that I take off from work until after my biopsy surgery the following week. After I was discharged later that evening, I was taken back home to rest. I didn't sleep very well that night because of the news I had just received. I couldn't wait any longer for my surgery date to come next week.

The day was finally here. March 28th, 2013. My biopsy surgery day. This day was the scariest and most dreadful day of my life. It seemed like it took forever to get to the hospital. I sat in the backseat of my Dad's truck alongside my Sister and my Mom. I felt so sick as we drove down the beltway headed to St. Agnes Hospital. It felt like we were hitting every bump in the road and it made me want to vomit. I was laying my head up against the window feeling weak and feeling like I was dying inside. I wanted to break down and cry, but I didn't want to cry in front of everyone.

After what seemed like forever, we finally arrived at the hospital. I could barely move from the back seat. My Mom went inside to get someone with a wheelchair to take me in. She came back with a technician and the wheelchair. The technician quickly began to push me inside to check in for my second and hopefully, negative biopsy surgery results. After I checked in, I waited a few minutes or so for someone to take me back for my surgery. I was a mess all over again and praying that it was nothing serious. I knew there was a strong possibility it was more than just nothing. One of the nurses came out to wheel me back to the exam room where I would prepare for surgery. After changing into a hospital gown, they prepped me with an IV and also took some blood. Once the nurse finished, I was lying there alone looking up at the ceiling thinking about so much in that moment. Like everything that has transpired leading up to this day.

A little while later, Dr. Henderson came in with my blood work results. He said that I have low red blood cells. I looked at him a bit confused but it also explains why I've been feeling weak and dizzy leading up to that day. Dr. Henderson explained that I would need a blood transfusion started before going into surgery. I personally didn't know very much about blood transfusions, but I have heard horror stories. So I asked several concerning questions about the transfusion to Dr. Henderson and he explained that I would be fine. Not long after our conversation, the surgical nurse came back into the room and started my blood transfusion. She also gave me some medication that would help suppress my coughing that I was still experiencing.

After I was prepped and ready for surgery, I was taken down to the surgical operating room where a team of technicians, nurses and Dr. Henderson was waiting. The Anesthesiologists started my anesthesia into my IV and moments later, I slowly fell off to sleep. I was awakened by the surgery staff yelling out my name like I remembered from my previous surgery back in December. This time was a little different. It was much scarier! I woke up having a massive panic attack. I couldn't breathe and I felt like I was going to die right there on the operating table! The medical staff started to give me oxygen to help me catch my breath but it didn't seem to work. I didn't know what was happening and thought something went horribly wrong during surgery causing me to have this attack. After a few attempts with giving me oxygen which felt like eternity, they were finally able to get my breathing under control. I was then taken into recovery. As I was lying there, all I could think about was my biopsy results. Again I was trying to remain hopeful but I couldn't help but wonder. The recovery nurse came back to talk to me. She explained that I would have to stay over for a few days to receive more blood transfusions. This was also to guarantee that I was closely monitored. I asked her about my test results. She explained that Dr. Henderson will come to my assigned hospital room once I am admitted to speak with me further about my surgery results. I said ok and then she proceeded to walk away.

My family was out in the waiting room. They thought that I was going to come out. Since I'm staying over, they were all taken up to my assigned room. I was told that I would be staying for the next few days. After about 45 minutes in recovery, I was transferred to my room on the 5th floor by a hospital technician. When the technician rolled my bed into the room, my family was awaiting my arrival, and for my biopsy results as well. After getting settled into my hospital room bed, I just laid there trying to talk a little with my family. Since having my neck cut open, it wasn't easy. I had a white gauze taped across my neck over my surgical scar. I was in some pain but with all the medication given to me during surgery, it wasn't too bad at that specific moment. I was feeling nervous about what could possibly happen once Dr. Henderson came to see me. After what seemed like forever, Dr. Henderson came into the room and greeted everyone. Next, he went on to share my life changing news. He said that I had Cancer. Hodgkin Lymphoma to be exact... On this day, Thursday March 28th, 2013, my entire life was changed...forever.

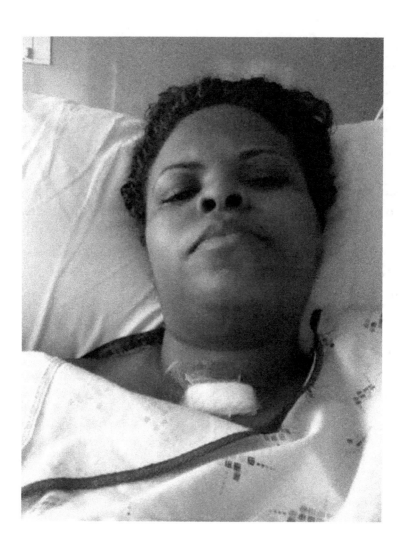

Chapter 4:
The Journey To Survival

*T*he news took me and my family by storm. I didn't know how to think or feel. I was truly broken and afraid. To hear the word "Cancer" was like someone hearing their fate in court in front of a judge giving them to the "Death Sentence". Dr. Henderson continued as he explained that there was a cancer center connected to the hospital just below us. He told us that I would speak with an oncology doctor to talk more about my treatment options to fight this life threatening disease. He said that he would see me for a follow up appointment in a few weeks to check my neck. After that he left the room. When he left out I wanted to break down into tears. I held back. I wanted to be strong. I couldn't cry in front of my family. I had to do my best to hold it together for myself, and them as well. Trying my best to hide it on the outside, but within I was feeling so many mixed emotions. I felt like my life as I knew it, was taken away from me in just a few short hours. I knew leading up to this day that there was a big possibility but to hear it come to life, was so real.

My family stayed for a little while longer as we all took in this new and devastating news. Then they left early that evening and I was left alone to soak in my tears. Pain and hurt is what I strongly recall after taking in a word that I so dreaded hearing. I knew this was going to change my life in a way that I couldn't even fathom at the time. As I said I was prepared as I knew how to be at that point for this sort of situation. I hoped that it all worked in my favor, but I also knew it would be challenging. So at that moment I was distraught. I honestly just wanted to be left alone. I needed a minute to think. Every so often the cancer unit shift nurse would come check on me. She needed to check my vitals. There was just a feeling of sadness that I didn't need everyone to be there to see. But I knew that they were only doing their job.

A few days went by and I haven't really talked to anyone about my new diagnosis. I was still trying to cope. There was so much that I learned so quickly. It was still a lot to manage for myself so I wasn't so ready to share just yet. I only confided in a couple close friends. For the most part, I kept the news to myself. It was my last day at the hospital and before I was discharged, my new oncology doctor, Dr. Mills came by my room. We sat and discussed what the next steps were for my new journey to cancer survival. Dr. Mills assured me that I would be given the best treatments to beat this cancer battle. I was also told that I would be given several treatment options. We spoke for a while and set a date to have my power port procedure. This procedure would allow me to start receiving chemotherapy in a week. After that she left. Next the staff nurse came in. She had my discharge papers. She explained to me that I would be given the final ok to leave shortly by the cancer unit doctor. I called my Mom and told her that I would be free to go home soon. She said that she and my Dad would be on their way to pick me up.

A few hours went by and just as she said, they were both ready to bring me home. I got dressed and prepared to leave. The unit doctor came to see me briefly. Then I was given the thumbs up to be discharged from the hospital. I was happy about going home. I left there feeling like I had a ton of weights on my shoulders. It seemed as if my mind was running one hundred miles. I had so many things to get in order. At the same time, I couldn't stop worrying. I needed to schedule my power port surgery. I wanted to start receiving chemotherapy treatments as soon as possible. I also needed to call my supervisor to let him know about my new diagnosis. I need them to know that I would be out of work for a while.

I was thinking a lot, crying often throughout that day and just sitting around at home. So much had transpired over the last few days while I was admitted in the hospital. I couldn't quite understand why God chose me to go through this. To be honest, I was very upset with the thought of it all. It had my mind bothered as I couldn't seem to snap out of my thoughts. I just couldn't process it. The next morning, I scheduled my power port surgery for the following week. I was still feeling very sick and coughing persistently. It was now April 2013. I received visits from close friends and family. Having their company during this down time really meant a lot. I lived alone, so I truly appreciated each and every one of them. I didn't want to be alone. Everything was still unreal and too much thinking wasn't good for me.

A week has gone by and it was the day of my power port procedure. It was starting to be my new reality. It was time to get this object placed into the right side of my chest in a few hours. My parents came to pick me up. They were going to drive me back to St. Agnes Hospital where the surgery would take place. While we were driving up the highway I just sat in the backseat thinking a lot. We arrived an hour later, and we all walked into the surgical department so that I could do the usual check in routine. Then I took a seat and waited to be called back for surgery. My sitting time was very short lived. I was called back by one of the surgical nurses. I walked with her to a room where I would change, have my vitals checked and an IV put into my arm. Not long after, I was escorted to my suite for the hour. I laid on the hard, cold table while the surgery staff was prepping. Thankfully one of the surgical technicians put a warm blanket over my body to keep me warm and comfortable. For this particular operation, I didn't have to receive full general anesthesia. Instead I was given local anesthesia where I am still awake during the procedure.

As I was lying there, I felt the anesthesia kicking into my IV. I was sedated and the surgical doctor proceeded to cut open the right side of my upper chest right above my breast with a tiny incision. Then he took a few moments to find my main vein connected to my heart. After that he proceeded to cut a bigger incision right below to insert the power port. I felt the tugging and pressure but very little pain. After about 45 minutes or so, the surgery was over and I was now ready to be taken into recovery. While sitting there, I was thinking about everything life altering for me and my family from this point on. I'd gone through so much. But I realized far more important than that, I made it through so much. After clearing out of the recovery, I was able to return home. The only thing left to do at the moment, was to wait on a date to see Dr. Mills for another follow up appointment. Then I would be able to begin my first round of treatments. Little did I know the roller coaster ride was just getting started.

Chapter 5:

I Knew I Disliked Roller Coaster Rides

*A*fter being home a few days after having power port surgery, I noticed a strange spot right below my lower abdominal area. I also noticed the same strange spot on my leg. I couldn't help but to worry and sent a picture of both spots via text to my oncology doctor, Dr. Mills. She responded back asking that I contact my primary doctor about the spots. I called the office of my primary physician to make an appointment to have them looked at. I was scheduled for the next day. When I went to visit and have the spots tested, she couldn't explain what or where the marks came from. She advised that I will receive my results via the patient online portal within a few days and then we could discuss further to treat if necessary. I left the doctor's office and went back home to wait for the next few days on my results. It was the third day since my appointment and my results were finally in. The results showed that I had a staph infection called MRSA (Methicillin-resistant Staphylococcus aureus). I didn't have a clue what that was so of course I googled it. This news also explained why I was having terrible pain with my power port. I noticed before the MRSA results that my port wasn't healing properly. It was painful to the touch. With this new diagnosis, I had to go into the cancer center to have the port looked at by my oncology doctor's nurse. I called my Dad and told him that I had an emergency appointment scheduled for the following day at the cancer center. I was concerned about this MRSA diagnosis now. Reading up on it made matters worse. The following day, my Dad took me to St. Agnes Cancer Center. After I checked in, I was taken back for vitals and to be seen by Nurse Kathy. As I was sitting in the treatment center, it truly amazed me. It was my first time seeing firsthand what a cancer center looked like up close and in person.

Nurse Kathy proceeded to wipe my chest area where my power port is inserted with alcohol. She had to because she needed to take some blood. When she went to stick the needle into my chest, I jumped and yelled out in so much pain. Nurse Kathy noticed my painful reaction and knew right away that something was wrong with my port. She walked away to speak with Dr. Mills. She made the decision to keep me. She wanted to begin treating me with antibiotics for the Staph Infection. Nurse Kathy had to take blood from my arm the old fashion way. After running my blood test, the results showed that my platelet count was very low. Not only was I going to receive antibiotics for the Staph Infection, but I was going to receive some blood transfusions to up my platelet counts as well. I was extremely exhausted and it was only the beginning. After talking with Dr. Mills about my admission, I called and told my Dad that I wasn't going back home because they wanted to admit me. Shortly after, a hospital technician came to take me to the cancer unit where I would be staying for a few days or so.

One day went by. Then two days went by. I was still having night sweats which made my stay uncomfortable. I was repeatedly having to call the nurse for new gowns and bedding often. As soon as I closed my eyes to get some rest, I burst into these extreme cold sweats. The cancer unit nurse wasn't bothered by me. She told me that it was her job to take care of me. But in my mind it was irritating and uncomfortable because I was used to taking care of myself. After she left for the hundredth time, I laid there thinking and began to have a very bad melt down. An anxiety attack is what most would call it. I have never experienced a moment like this before. It was like the devil was over my body holding me down. I couldn't get him off of me. I cried out while pressing the nurse's station button to get some help. The staff nurse came back into my room asking what was wrong. I couldn't do anything but cry. I felt so embarrassed because I didn't like to cry in front of others. She made me feel comfortable by telling me that I will be ok. Then she gave me some medication into my IV to help me rest. Within minutes, I was fast asleep. When I woke back up later that evening, I felt better. It seemed as if I hadn't had any rest for months. I was happy that I was somewhat rested after that scary melt down episode. I laid there for a little while before falling back to sleep until the next morning. Not long after I woke up, the café server came into my room at 7am with breakfast. I was able to enjoy some good food, finally. For months my stomach was so upset and I had no appetite. I was excited that I was able to eat.

By the third day in the hospital receiving antibiotics, they moved my IV into three or four different locations in my arm. The antibiotics were so strong that it was causing my veins to blowout. My platelet count wasn't going up. Because of this I was receiving rounds and rounds of blood transfusions, and antibiotics at the same time. Now that Dr. Mills discovered this issue, she decided to replace the IV with a PICC (Peripherally inserted central catheter) line. It needed to be placed in my arm to finish up the MRSA treatment. Two PICC line technicians came into my room a few hours later to do just that. It was very painful! I was lying there in my hospital bed as if I was Jesus up on the cross. I had my arms stretched out while they inserted the thick tube lining into my right arm that went into my vein. This experience was hell. After the quick and painful measure, the technicians left my room. I waited for a nurse to come back to start another round of antibiotics. I had hopes that this time I didn't have any issues with my count.

The next day I was lying in my hospital bed watching television. I was having some pain with my power port so I decided to lift the gauze up to take a look. I couldn't believe my eyes. There was a green colored discharge coming out of my chest where the port was. I immediately called for a nurse to come take a look at it. When the nurse came in to check, right away she looked surprised. She told me that she couldn't explain why I was experiencing this discharge. She said that she would go call someone for further direction on what to do. Not long after, she returned stating that I would need to have an emergency surgery. The port had to be removed as soon as possible. It was pretty scary. A couple hospital technicians came to take me down to have this emergency surgery.

After it was complete, I was returned to my room to rest and to continue my transfusions. My blood count still wasn't up like they were hoping. Dr. Mills came up to see me the next day. She explained that she had spoken with a colleague over at another hospital facility for some direction. She needed more clarity on how to get my platelet counts up in order to start my chemotherapy treatments. Her colleague told her to give me a round of transfusions, and one round of chemo before I was discharged to see what happens. Dr. Mills did what he advised and to our surprise, that actually worked. My platelet counts shot up to a good number. We were both excited, but that was short-lived because soon we would discover another issue.

The next day while sitting in bed, I began to experience this burning sensation under my right thigh. I went to touch the area where the burning was coming from and noticed a bumpy round sore. I called for the nurse and when she came in, I showed her the sore. She called down to the cancer center for the nurse practitioner to come up. Her name was Erin. She came up to my room to look at the sore as well and also took pictures to send to Dr. Mills. Dr. Mills came back with yet another diagnosis for me- the sore was shingles! Now we had to start treating it before I was released from the hospital. I tell you, I was going through some strange things with my immune system being weak. It was getting to be very overwhelming.

The following day, a staff doctor and her assistant came into my room to talk to me about performing a bone marrow biopsy. I had absolutely no idea what that was. I wasn't prepared for what came next. The doctor explained that the procedure would take all of 15-30 minutes to perform. First she would numb my hip area. Then she would use a long needle to insert through my hip bone to remove bone marrow. This test was performed to see if the cancer had spread into my bone marrow. I was in so much pain during that procedure. I wanted to hop off the bed and run but her assistant was there to hold my hands through the process. My family was also visiting at the time. They were asked to step out of the room so that they could perform the procedure. When they l returned I was in so much pain, I just wanted to be alone, so not long after, my family left for the evening. The following day another doctor and his assistant came into my room. I was looking at the both of them with an expression of confusion. It seemed like there was always someone new coming into my room to see me for something. He said that the previous doctor from yesterday did not take enough bone marrow, and that he had to perform the test again. I couldn't believe what I was hearing. I was mortified. But what choice did I have? So I laid there to have the painful test done all over again. I told them to make sure it was done properly this time. It felt like he was digging into my hip forever to get enough bone marrow. I was crying and praying that it was over soon. He was finally finished with the procedure in what felt like eternity. I was angry but also thinking, "I hope that it was enough bone marrow removed this time or else this was the last try."

A few days, later after a couple rounds of chemo, I was free to go home.

It was coming up on Memorial Day weekend. I was not feeling well but I was pushing through. They wanted to give my first port womb some time to heal before moving forward. They had to decide whether or not to replace it again right there, or to the other side of my chest. So I went on about my life with a PICC line still hanging from my arm.

It was Sunday May 26, 2013, the Sunday before Memorial Day. I woke up that morning and my arm felt strange. It felt numb as if no blood was circulating where my PICC line was. I was worried thinking maybe I slept on it through the night. I was advised not to or there was a chance of getting a blood clot. I went on about my day to a barbeque with family to enjoy myself. In the back of my mind all I could think about was the possibility. I tried my best to hide it with a smile. Although deep down inside my thoughts were scattered, I didn't worry too much because I wanted to have a good day with family.

Later that evening after I returned back home, I made a call to my oncology doctor. She didn't answer so I left a message on her voicemail. I decided to rest because I wasn't feeling too well. A few minutes later Dr. Mills called me back telling me that I needed to come up to St. Agnes Hospital, or go to a closer hospital to have my arm looked at. I got back up and got dressed to head down to Southern Maryland Hospital to get looked at. When I arrived and checked in, I was praying for a positive outcome. I didn't want to be admitted overnight. Well that is exactly what happened. I did have a blood clot in my right arm where the PICC line was, so I had no choice but to stay. I was so upset.

After I was admitted and transferred to my room that I shared with another patient affected by MRSA, the unit nurse came to check my vitals. She had to explain that my PICC line would be removed shortly. I asked her if the process would be painful. She responded quite snappy that it wouldn't be as if I wasn't the patient in pain, and living with cancer. I returned her attitude with one of my own; giving her a mean look as she turned to walk out. After she walked away to get the tools needed to remove my PICC line, I went onto YouTube to see how the procedure would go. I was curious because it hurt while being put in. But after watching a video, I felt at ease. It was reassuring to see that it wouldn't be painful while being removed.

The snappy nurse returned moments later and by this point it was a little after midnight. I made the mistake of telling her that I looked up a video and felt at ease knowing that it wouldn't hurt. Do you know that this crazy lady was upset that I decided to do that? I just gave her yet another look that made her more than aware that I was 100% convinced that she was crazy, lol. She proceeded to unscrew the ends of the PICC line. Then she slowly pulled it out of my arm with ease. That was it. Next she gave me some medication for the pain. After that she left the room. Within the next few moments I started to feel weird from the medication. I began to sweat profusely and then the medication knocked me out. The next day I explained to the morning nurse how the medication made me feel and she told the doctor. The unit doctor decided to give me a bracelet to wear showing that I could no longer receive those pills again.

The next couple days were not pleasant. I was feeling so miserable in that hospital. I cried every day that I was in there. Although friends and family came to visit, I still felt alone and miserable. It was nothing like my stay at St. Agnes Hospital. The staff wasn't too welcoming, nor did they check on me very much. I contacted Dr. Mills to see if she could send a helicopter or something to get me out of there. I didn't eat anything besides the food my family and good girlfriend brought for me. I didn't watch any television either. I just found myself sleeping and praying to be released soon. I cried silently so much. I didn't want to bother my roommate. She was miserable as well. After talking with her briefly, she told me that she left one bad hospital from just giving birth, only to come to another unpleasant hospital. If that wasn't enough, she also had to have a staph infection as well. We were both suffering.

After asking to see the lead doctor several times, on the third day he finally came to see me. Of course I was beyond upset with this entire process by then. He spoke with my oncology doctor over the phone. After their call he explained that I needed to stay at least one more day. I wasn't happy with the news but I had no choice. I wanted to make sure my arm was ok. He left my room and as I laid there in bed for another long day in the hospital, I found some comfort in listening to music. The next day the lead doctor came in to speak with me again before I was freed. He explained that I will have to give myself shots of blood thinner called Lovenox every day into my stomach. I was looking at him traumatized by what he was directing me to do. I felt my life was in a whirlwind. I left that hospital and almost ran off to my car happy to leave that hell of a place. I was also sad that all of this was happening to me. I was really upset to have a blood clot in my arm. When I got home that afternoon I ate like crazy. I was on steroids for a couple weeks now. They were prescribed by my oncology doctor so it gave me one big appetite. After eating something I laid down to rest a bit from these crazy past few days. Every night after felt long because I couldn't rest well. So many thoughts going through my mind, my night sweats were still going on, and I was slightly coughing. Luckily it wasn't as often as before. So I had to make my restless nights work the best I could.

My Mom was here with me most nights to look after me since I lived alone. I was thankful that she was. One late evening I woke up to use the restroom. While I was in there I began to experience this really sharp pain in my legs. I felt them lock. The pressure was insane. I didn't want to scream out to my Mom for help and alarm her, but I wasn't fully dressed and had no other option because I couldn't move my legs. I tried falling off the toilet onto the floor and crawling back to my bed. The pain was unbearable. It was at least 3am and my Mom was downstairs sound asleep. After a few calls out to her, she finally answered. She came up to assist me back to my bed. I couldn't explain what exactly had just happened. I waited until morning to contact my oncology doctor's office to tell them. I was advised to come into the cancer center for observation. I also spoke with one of my Aunts who is a nurse. She told me that it sounded like muscle spasms. She said that I needed to get some bananas to get my potassium levels up. Later that day one of my good girlfriends came over with some bananas and muscle cream. She assisted by rubbing the cream on my knees and legs. It was to give me some pain relief. At this point it seemed to be I discovered a new ailment every day. Now add on the fact that I had to give myself blood thinner shots in my stomach each day until after my treatments were completed "stressed" was an understatement. It was a really dreadful storm in my life.

Chapter 6:
Stage 4

A few days later I was scheduled for another appointment with my oncology doctor to have my blood checked. She also needed to check to see how my power port scar was healing. At this appointment, Dr. Mills would decide the next steps to continue my treatments. She explained that we would move forward replacing the power port on the left side of my chest. Then we'd schedule bi weekly chemotherapy treatments. In that meeting I was reminded to ask what stage my cancer was in. She said that I was a Stage 4. It was like I was hit with a ton of bricks to my face. Dr. Mills then assured me that Hodgkin Lymphoma even at Stage 4, is highly curable. I still didn't hear what she was saying clearly. I was more scared about my chances of survival. After my appointment with Dr. Mills, I left the cancer center more terrified than usual because of the news I just received. When I returned home, I contacted the scheduling department to make an appointment to have the second port put in. The surgery was scheduled for the following week.

The day of the surgery was like any other surgery day. I was filled with anxiety and praying for a successful outcome. I was thinking to myself, "What if I get a staph infection again?" Then I thought "What if I don't heal quickly enough to continue my chemotherapy treatments?" All of the what if's were running through my mind at that time while I waited to go back for surgery. A few hours later, my new power port was placed on the left side of my chest, and I was headed back home to rest and prepare to start my third round of chemotherapy treatments the following week.

I had a lot of time to think, and personal business to also take care of while home. I took a short term disability while off from work. I needed some other means of income to help me pay my bills. I reached out to several organizations that were provided to me by my social worker at the cancer center. Organizations like The Leukemia and Lymphoma Society and Lymphoma Research Foundation. They helped me with financial assistance without a problem. It was one less burden of many that I was dealing with at this time.

As the days were passing me by, I was thinking about the part of this journey that I was about to endure. Family and good friends came to visit me often. I was truly going through so many obstacles so I appreciated the visits. I was still faulting the man (God) above for this difficult time, but I knew deep inside that he didn't make mistakes when he chose me to go through this. Of course it took lots of prayer and understanding to realize that. I just celebrated my 28th birthday on May 8th but it wasn't the same this year because of my sickness. However, I was grateful to see another birthday despite my battle with cancer.

It was the day to start my third chemo treatment. I was now sitting in my new home at the St. Agnes Cancer Center scheduled for bi weekly chemotherapy treatments for 6 months and 12 rounds. As I sat in the treatment chair, the nurse wiped my chest where the power port is. She said to me, "Count out loud to three and take deep breaths." Then she stuck the needle in through my chest into the port. I was going to experience this routine every single time for chemo treatments. It wasn't a pleasant experience. I figured eventually I would get used to it. I asked the nurse if in the future I requested an ice pack to help numb that area would it be ok. She said that it can be arranged. The nurse took some blood and then began my treatments. Since I was having breathing issues due to weakened lungs, I was only going to receive Adriamycin, Vinblastine and Dacarbazine (AVD) chemotherapy treatments, and not the full ABVD treatment. The Bleomycin regimen would hurt my lungs more. As I sat there receiving my round of treatment, I listened to music to relax my mind. My parents were also there waiting for me. I would always need someone to drive me to and from treatments.

Three treatments down and I'm actually feeling ok besides the fatigue. When I returned home later in the afternoon, I drank lots of fluids and got some rest. The next few days were a little different. One day I woke up feeling really drained and could barely function. I called the after-hours emergency line and explained my symptoms. The service representative asked me to come in once the office opens to be checked out. Once I hung up the phone, I called my Dad to ask if he could take me to the cancer center. A few hours later he came to pick me up from my home to take me. We arrived at the cancer center and after checking in, I was taken to get checked out by a nurse. She took some blood as I waited. When my results came back it wasn't a positive result. My white blood count was low, and I was experiencing tingling in my legs. Oh joy, something else to add to my growing list of things wrong. I was feeling really weak, so Dr. Mills decided to admit me for a day or two. She wanted to keep a close eye on me. I called and told my Dad to come back so that I could tell him what just transpired.

I was laying in my hospital bed (once again) that evening thinking about a good meal. The steroids that I was on made me want to eat up everything in sight. Before I was diagnosed, I wanted a good meal from my good girlfriend's grandmother. She made this really tasty baked chicken and rice dish that I loved. I got very sick before I could get it fixed. So, I asked my Mom (who also cooks very well) to fix me a nice meal like it was Thanksgiving. The next evening, she came up to the hospital to stay with me and boy did she deliver! She brought me: baked chicken, greens, yams, and rice to enjoy. I was very hungry often in the hospital because the times for dining always seemed weird (serving breakfast at 7am, lunch at 11am and dinner at around 4pm). Couple that with me being on steroids and I suddenly became a glutton. The nurses thought giving me graham crackers and Jell-O would fix my hunger, but it didn't! It only pissed me off. So, I was extremely grateful to and for my Mom on this day, with all of this amazing food. But this story would not be mine without some sort of inconvenience, right? When I went to eat my food, I couldn't taste the flavors. I was so devastated and pushed the food tray across the room away from me. I started to cry. My Mom was sitting in the chair next to my bed and looked at me with concern. She asked me what was wrong. I told her that I couldn't taste my food. At that moment I then realized that my taste buds were fading away. I knew then that everything that I was going through was truly real. Even more than I thought before. I was over being in the hospital. I wanted to go home to my own bed. I was feeling lonely and miserable because so much was happening all at once. And oh yeah, I was STILL hungry!

When I woke up the next morning, the food service brought in my breakfast, and I did my best to eat some food although I could not taste anything at all. After I ate I just laid around watching the television until it was time to go. By early afternoon I was giving the "ok" to go home. I was so ecstatic! I was just hoping I was able to stay home longer this time without something else happening.

It was the middle of June and it was really hot out. I wanted to enjoy my summer despite my tough battle with cancer. I was still out of work because of the complications that I continued to experience. Every time I thought I was ready to go back, something else happened to me. So I decided that I would be ready after the 4th of July weekend. After going in and out of the hospital, up and downs, happy days, sad days and anything else you could name, I was ready to go back to work. I was scheduled to have my second PET scan performed to see where my cancer was at this point. To God be the glory my scan showed zero signs of the cancer cells like before. I was truly amazed because it was only a short time since the start of receiving treatments. But after meeting with Dr. Mills, she stated that the scan was accurate-whew, a blessing. Despite the improvement in my scans, I would still need to complete my treatments until the end of the last round. That news burst my little happy bubble. I thought in my mind that I could be done with all of this because my scans were clear. That wasn't the case.

It was time to return back to work. It was the Tuesday after the Independence Holiday weekend. Everyone was happy to see me back at work. One of my colleagues and friends often shared with me that so many people were asking about me. They wanted to know where I was. Not many people at my workplace knew that I was out sick with cancer. So once I returned back, I told some of them about my diagnosis. Those that I spoke to about it were really shocked. However, they were also very happy that I was doing well and pushing through my journey.

Getting back into the swing of things wasn't easy but I was determined to make it through. I was continuing my bi-weekly chemotherapy treatments like clockwork, and my job even allowed me to take off on those treatment days. I was scheduled to finish up my treatments in September and I COULD NOT WAIT. The celebration of life after cancer was near. I often thought a lot about what life would be like after I was done with my daily back and forth visits to the cancer center/hospital. After what felt like a never-ending cycle of body ailments, new diagnoses, failed tests, confusion, anger, pain, fear, etc., I was thrilled to be so close to the finish line.

Chapter 7:
To the Finish Line

*I*t was Friday September 27, 2013. That was my final day of chemotherapy treatments. All I could say was, "Won't he do it?" I was beyond excited. Six months, twelve rounds, a blood clot, low platelet counts, shingles, a staph infection, in and out of the hospital, and countless days filled with ups and downs. I thank God for seeing me through it all. He heard my cry. He saved me from this life threatening disease. I went through the storm on fire but ready to overcome it all. That's exactly what I did. Perseverance got me to the finish line.

I was at the Cancer Center with my parents ready to rock and roll with this last treatment. I had on my best outfit for this day. Like any other treatment day, I was prepped by one of the center nurses and ready to receive my chemotherapy. I was still feeling sick from the previous treatment two weeks ago. The upset stomach started around my fifth or sixth cycle. The sickness from the treatments started to make my stomach sour. I always felt as if I needed to vomit. The feeling was miserable. After every cycle I was so ill. It just wouldn't let up. On top of everything else I still couldn't taste the foods that I was eating. By the time it was time for my next treatment two weeks later, I didn't feel any better. But despite the ill feeling I was having, I was happy for this day. The nurse started my chemo treatment. Then Dr. Mills came in to talk with me. She wanted to see how I was feeling about it being my last day and overcoming such a tough journey. I told her that I was blessed to have her in my life. I was joyful for this moment. After we talked a bit, she walked away. Within the same breath there I was receiving treatment for the last time. I was thinking about how I couldn't wait to ring the "Last Day of Chemo" bell at the end.

An hour or so later I completed my last round of 12 chemotherapy treatments. The center's nurse came back to flush my power port with saline solution. Then he removed the needle from my chest. Before he walked away, my parents and I took pictures with him. I knew for a fact my Mom and Dad were ecstatic for this day as much as I was. We then walked over to the bell where Dr. Mills was standing alongside her assistant Nurse Kathy. I grabbed the string to the bell and rang that bell so hard. It almost came off the wall. That should tell you how gratified I was in that very moment. I hugged Dr. Mills and Nurse Kathy. I thanked them for all that they've done for me over the past six months. The team at the cancer center of St. Agnes was always so pleasant and caring with all my needs. I was very thankful to have them as my cancer treatment center.

I checked out with the receptionist and then my parents and I walked out still filled with so much joy. As we were approaching the car, I looked down and saw a stack of money lying there on the ground. You would have thought after having treatment that I wouldn't be able to move so quickly to grab it but I did. Can you believe it was over $700? My Dad said to me, "It's probably more on the other side of the other vehicle." He was right, there was more. It was $40 more that peeled away from the stack of money that I was holding in my hands. My Mom was sitting behind me in the back seat. I told them that it wouldn't be right if we didn't find out if the money was reported to someone at the front desk. My mom and I went back inside. We checked with the receptionist to see if anyone had mentioned anything. She told us no and then I asked the receptionist to take down my number. I wanted her to contact me if anyone decided to report their money missing. My Mom and I walked back to the car. After that we left. I was thinking to myself on the ride home that I would give it a week for someone to claim the money. If not, I will take this as a blessing from God. Not only was it my last day of chemo treatment after a long survival journey, but I was blessed with lots of money. It was my lucky Friday.

Part 2

Chapter 8:

A Second Chance

*I*t's time to find my new leaf on life as I continue to celebrate my "Cancer Free" self. It was October 2013, a month after my final chemotherapy treatment and I was beginning to find level grounds in my life. I planned a getaway trip to Puerto Rico with one of my friends. So, as you can guess, no one ever called to claim that money, but I digress, lol. I couldn't be more excited to get away for a few days to let my hair down. I mean, after the rollercoaster ride I endured 12 months or so, I was ready to have some fun under the sun. I shopped for some cute summer dresses and swimsuits. I could not wait. A few weeks went by and it was time to fly out to beautiful Puerto Rico. Before I knew it my girlfriend and I were checking in at the airport and ready to take flight. We arrived a few hours later safely in Puerto Rico.

We got settled into our hotel room. Then we got changed into our swimsuits to go have a good time out on the beach. After we changed of course we had to take some cute pictures like most women do, lol. After posing for several photos, we headed out the door. We wanted to find a good place to eat and have a drink. We walked around until we came up on a nice tiki bar and restaurant that sat across from the beach. We stepped inside as the host greeted us both and led us to our table. The restaurant was really neat with Caribbean style décor and Caribbean sounds playing in the background. The waiter came over to take our orders. As she concluded we took the time to take in the atmosphere. It was a joy. We were surrounded by a few others that all seemed to be enjoying themselves as well.

After we ate our food and enjoyed our drinks, we headed for the beach to relax. We found a spot to lay out with our rented chairs and umbrella. They did their job making sure to shade us from the sun. As I'm lying out on the beach reflecting over a nice cocktail, I begin thinking back to the past 12 months of my life. It was a very trying period but the battle against cancer taught me how to fight in a whole different way. I didn't lose hope and even through my adversities, I chose not to give up. My girlfriend and I were having a good ole time with lots of laughter and fun. We laid on the beach for a couple hours just watching the other beach goers.

After some time out on the beach we headed back to the room to shower and change. Our plan was to go out on the town to enjoy the nightlife. Once we headed back out, we found a nice lounge a few blocks away from our hotel. It was packed with so many beautiful people. The D.J. was playing all the hottest hits. We had a blast. After a couple hours and lots of dancing, we made our way back to the hotel to get some rest. Our goal was to do it all over again the next day, and take advantage of tourist activities in town.

Unfortunately, all good things come to an end. After days of sun, sand and sangria, it was finally our last day in Puerto Rico, and we wanted to go out with a bang. We took a tour of Old San Juan and also went shopping. Then we enjoyed some delicious food in town. After that we headed back for our afternoon spa hour at the hotel resort. As I was enjoying my massage, I was thinking about the next steps to come when I returned back home. I still had my monthly appointments with my oncology doctor, returning to working full time, and overall back to reality of the fully recovered lifestyle. "What's next?" That was my new biggest question to myself.

After my return from Puerto Rico, I planned a big party to celebrate my survival with Cancer. I invited my close friends and family and we had such a blast. Great music, food and much needed laughter filled the room.

Then I worked steadfastly to establish a new normal. I was often going through moments where I wasn't feeling my best. I felt like although I was cancer free, I was still going through the motions of trauma. I didn't look like myself either. I had these scars that were left behind from the many surgeries I received throughout my battle. I gained weight from the steroids. My hair was severely thin from shedding over the months of treatment that I received. Here it was December 2013, and I made the craziest decision I could ever make. I decided to go to the beauty salon to cut my hair off. Well what was left of it anyway. I was so scared to do it because I was used to having long pretty hair my entire life. I needed to make this change to get my hair back to good health again. So I did it. I went for the big chop.

I called a beautician that a friend referred to me and made this life altering appointment. I was scheduled for a few days later. I was both excited and nervous. When I arrived at the salon, I took a few minutes and sat in my vehicle before going inside. I didn't know if I was making the right decision but I was here now. There wasn't any turning back. I got out of my car and walked up to the salon. Once I got in I instantly admired the décor. You could tell that the owner had some great interior taste. I was greeted by a lady asking if I was Erica. I replied "Yes" and then she introduced herself as Del, my beautician. I said

"Hello" and then she took me back to her station. She asked me what I was in for. I told her that I wanted to chop all of my hair off but I was afraid of the outcome. Del assured me that I would look fine and suggested that I do it to bring my hair back to life again. She laughed at me because I kept making scary faces. Nevertheless, I was up for the change, so we did it. To my surprise, I loved it. My hair curled up really pretty (Although I believe it's because of the cancer treatments) and it was beautiful. At first I was afraid that once she turned that chair around that I would look crazy. Thankfully it was the total opposite. It was perfect.

Fast forward to January; it was the New Year and I was a new me! Taking things one day at a time to rebuild and (inadvertently) rebrand myself. I joined a workout movement to get this post cancer weight off of my body from taking steroids. I have to say I truly enjoyed it. I was coming up on my one-year survival anniversary and I wanted to celebrate in a big way. I decided to make it memorable with a spectacular photoshoot. So I found a great photographer to shoot with. He set the date and time, and it was up to me to find the perfect look and makeup artist. I had never done a photoshoot before so this was totally new for me, but I was so eager about it and I did not want to let myself nor this photographer down.

It was now the day of my shoot and I was a bit antsy because I wanted my visuals to be exemplary. I decided that I wanted behind the scene footage to capture the moment. My friend helped me with a videographer. I arrived at the location of my shoot and everyone was there waiting for me. My makeup artist totally understood my vision through the detail of my makeover. Her work was phenomenal. The photographer was amazing as well. He made me feel very comfortable and I felt so glamorous. The shoot was a success. I could not wait to reveal them to the world on my anniversary day.

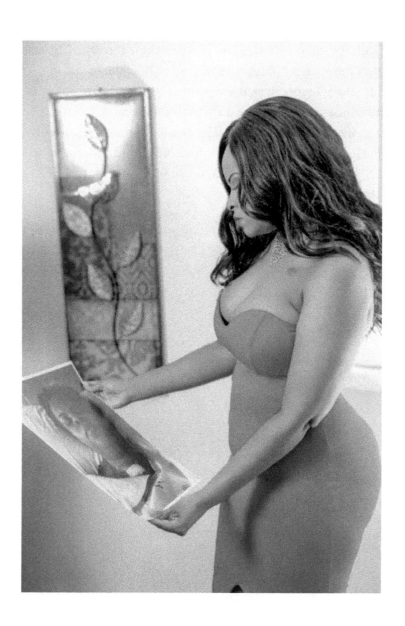

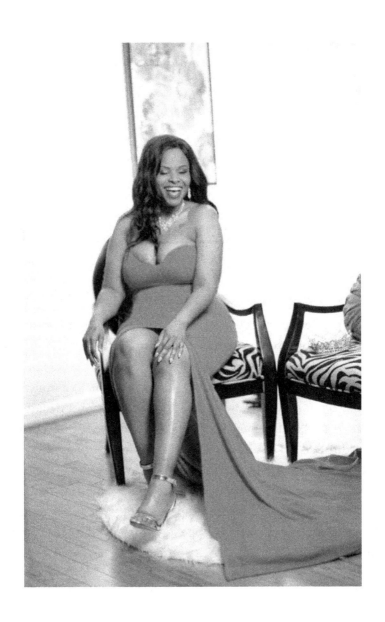

Chapter 9:

Walking For A Cause

After all, that I had endured and learned during this journey, and with a newfound, rejuvenated outlook on life, I decided to join the Lymphoma Research Foundation in their 5K Walk that was scheduled for April of 2014. I was thrilled to participate and give back to such a great cause. I reached out to family and friends to put together a walk and fundraiser team. I decided to call the team "Dzire2Survive". I even decided to create a purple team shirt that we all could wear to stand out. Purple symbolizes my ribbon color for Hodgkin's Lymphoma. I wanted this walk to be amazing. I also wanted it to be a fun time and an opportunity to express my gratitude as a survivor and now as an advocate. I wanted to give hope to others within the cancer community.

It was finally my one-year anniversary. It was a great feeling in every aspect. To think back to all that I overcame during my battle against cancer, I was filled with so much joy. I knew it was a blessing to have the opportunity to celebrate. The reflection of my life at this point was clear. I was truly blessed to have a second chance. I knew it was more life to live from here. I shared my beautiful photos with everyone on my social media pages. I received so much love. I decided to have an intimate dinner with those that supported me throughout my entire journey. My parents, , siblings, aunt, uncle, and a few of my closest loved ones were all there. I made private dinner reservations at PF Chang's Bistro (one of my favorite places to dine) and we had a good time and great conversation. I couldn't ask for anything better than to be side by side those that I love and also loved me.

On the day of the walk to raise awareness for lymphoma. I had on my purple tutu and purple bunny ears with my "Dzire2Survive" team shirt. I was super excited to be a part of an amazing organization for a great cause., and I was ready to hit the pavement. Over the last month my team raised a good sum of money for the walk. All of it would go back to help patients and their families affected by lymphoma. I have never done a walk or raised money before now. It felt good to do a good deed to help others. We arrived to the site at Chevy Chase Park in Chevy Chase, MD. We checked in and took pictures before it started as a team. The emcee said a few words before we took off for our 3 miles. All of the participants were having such a good time. There were so many teams of survivors, loved ones, and supporters here for the same cause.

We made it back to the finish line cheering away in excitement. The Lymphoma Research Foundation walk was a huge success. My team and I had such a blast. This was a time for the community to really come together. We did just that! We sent a message to all patients, survivors, and their families. That message was to "Never Give Up On Your Fight."

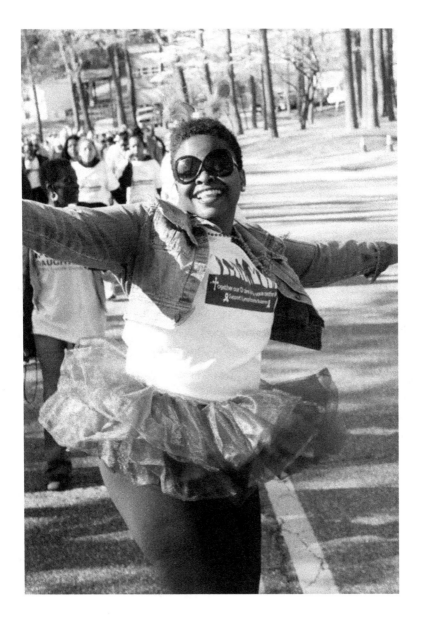

Chapter 10:
The 8ᵗʰ Day

*M*y 29th birthday was approaching on May 8th. Already a celebration of its own, I was even happier to celebrate while being cancer free. The previous year I felt alone and didn't celebrate my special day due to my illness. I had been dating someone special for a few months now, and I thought he was pretty great. He was caring, very open, and honest with me. He was also really patient, easy going, and handsome as well. He was always thinking of ways to make me smile, and I appreciate him for being a light in my life. When it came to my birthday, he went above and beyond. He thought it would be nice if we went away this year. I didn't want to do anything too big so we just traveled a few hours to a beautiful beach in New Jersey to relax. My man wanted to make sure my day was special from start to finish and he did an outstanding job. We traveled up to New Jersey on a beautiful Friday morning. The drive across bridges were particularly peaceful and enjoyable for me, as I love just taking short rides away from home just to get away.

When we arrived we checked into our Bed and Breakfast not too far from the water. We chose the perfect location for our stay. It was beautiful. The staff at the front desk were pleasant as they checked us in and gave directions to our room. After we got settled in and changed into some more relaxing clothes, we went out on the town to get a bite to eat. We hadn't eaten since breakfast before hitting the road. We found a small but nice café at the corner of the narrow street. They served both breakfast and lunch so we stopped off there. The hostess led us to a small table over by a window that looked out onto the street. We ordered some burgers and fries. We chatted about life and our future together. After we ate our food we agreed to go for a stroll. The warm spring breeze felt awesome as we walked along the sandy beach. We decided to go back to the room to get some rest before dinner later in the evening.

It was my big day. It was my birthday! The day was beautiful and I was truly blessed to see another year. He planned out a great day for me. I couldn't wait to see what was in store. We got up and got ready for a nice breakfast served right to the comfort of our room. I felt like a queen not having to lift one finger (well just to eat my food but that was about it, lol). After breakfast we enjoyed being lazy in bed with one another. After a few hours, we got dressed and headed out to the town. I wanted to do something fun so I found a bike rental place on the boardwalk. It wasn't a far walk from our bed and breakfast so we made our way there. It was early afternoon so there were people out enjoying their day. We arrived at the bike rental location and made our selections. I hadn't rode a bicycle in a very long time so it brought back memories from my childhood as a young girl riding throughout my neighborhood with friends. My boyfriend and I had a blast riding up and down the boardwalk passing by people. We did lots of sightseeing. We also liked grabbing bites to eat from food trucks parked on the boardwalk. . After about an hour of riding, we rode back to the bike rental location to return our bikes. Then we decided to walk around before heading back to get ready for my birthday dinner. We heard music coming from the pier. We went over to listen to the local band playing upbeat tunes for everyone to enjoy.

We went back to the room to prepare for dinner at a nice restaurant that he chose for my birthday celebration. I had my entire look in mind already. A cute black dress and some cute heels. I put them on and grinned from ear to ear. My new short black hair was cut perfectly. It was such a great look, and it definitely complimented my outfit. I stared at myself in the mirror and took it all in. "Yes, I feel like me. I look great!"

We left and headed out to the restaurant. The drive wasn't far from our hotel. The venue was very nice. It was an Italian cuisine. The atmosphere was beautiful with soft sounds of traditional Italian music playing in the background. The ambiance and the food were so delightful. I couldn't ask for anything better. He gifted me with a beautiful bracelet and teddy bear. I loved it so much. The night was perfect.

I enjoyed myself on my relaxing getaway. My boyfriend and I had such a peaceful and fun time with each other. I couldn't wait to see where our relationship was headed. I couldn't believe after such a roller coaster ride, I'd have so much peace. He's just so sweet and understanding of my needs. What more could I ask for?

I can actually say my life was on the right path. I was cancer free and now at this point I was seeing my oncology doctor once every three months. My follow up appointments were going great as well. I was blessed and happy to be in this space after such a roll coaster ride the year before. After my first walk with The Lymphoma Research Foundation (LRF), the organization was happy to share my life changing story on their "Story of Hope" page. Their mission is to eradicate lymphoma and serve those touched by this disease. I was honored to share my story and grateful for any life I was able to touch. I also started another great ambassador relationship with The Leukemia and Lymphoma Society (LLS). Their mission is to cure leukemia, lymphoma, Hodgkin's disease and myeloma. They also work to improve the quality of life of patients and their families. In essence, LLS exists to find cures and ensure access to treatments for blood cancer patients.   After I was newly diagnosed, I found out about these two amazing organizations. They were happy to assist myself and my family in any way possible. They supported me as a patient, survivor with financial assistance, and peer to peer support through their First Connection program.

Once I became cancer free, I decided to reach out to see how I could help support other newly diagnosed patients in need. Both LRF and LLS were very beneficial to me as their support helped me cope in such an incredible way.

Chapter 11:
No More Power In My Port

I was scheduled for my follow up appointment with Dr. Mills. As we were discussing my blood work results, we also discussed removing my power port. That was like sweet music to my ears. She wanted to schedule the surgery for the following month, in September. I was ecstatic to hear the good news. Plus, I no longer wanted to have that foreign object inside my chest any longer. I couldn't wait. After she checked for enlarged lymph nodes in her routine, we talked about my next appointment schedule and then I left the cancer center. I couldn't wait to share the news with my boyfriend and my family about having my port removed in a few weeks. Once I got to my car I called my boyfriend and even before he could ask about my appointment, I told him with excitement that I was given the thumbs up to have my port removed. He said, "That is great news to hear." After we were off the phone, I called and told my family the news as well. I drove home filled with absolute joy. This was a milestone in my life that I know many patients fighting cancer look forward to.

It was the morning of September 5th 2014, the day of my port removal surgery at St. Agnes Hospital. I woke up in tears and feeling very emotional. I had a bad dream that caused so many different feelings and thoughts. My boyfriend called out to me to wake me from my sleep. Once I was fully up, I couldn't stop crying. He just held me until I got myself together. He said that he heard me crying while asleep so he wanted to wake me to make sure that I was ok. I wasn't ok. I was thinking about my journey to get to this day. The ups, the downs and everything else in between. After a few moments of crying, I got up to shower and got dressed for my surgery appointment. I was really afraid. I couldn't eat or drink anything before surgery. That was ok because I wasn't in any mood to eat anyway.

We were on the road headed to the hospital. My Mom couldn't make it, so it was just my Dad and my boyfriend. I was having a bittersweet moment. It was just an overall strange feeling I was experiencing knowing what I've overcome over the past year and a half of my life. When we arrived at the hospital facility we parked and went into the front area. I checked in at the front desk. I sat for a few moments before being called back by one of the nurses to begin prepping for my surgery. I followed behind the nurse towards the back. When we got to one of the exam rooms and began prepping, the nurse took my vitals and proceeded to start an IV but she looked confused. I asked her what was wrong and she stated that she could not get a good vein. She tried my right arm but the same thing happened. After trying in another part of my right arm, the nurse said that she would have to put an IV in through the vein in my neck. I said, "Huh???!!" a bit confused by her statement. She asked if I'd been drinking enough water and I told her yes quite often. I was horrified to hear what had to be done in order to move forward with surgery. I didn't have any other choice if I wanted to have the port removed. The nurse stepped out and after a few moments she then returned. She started an IV through my neck. After doing so, she led me down to the surgical room. Like any other time when having my ports put in or taken out, I laid on the surgical table and waited for the local anesthesia to begin to sedate me. Then the surgeon began cutting the left side of my chest to remove the power port.

I couldn't wait until the surgeon was done so that I could get a picture of the object. It was a memory that I wanted to keep with me forever. It was another piece of this puzzle that I planned to piece all together. I was almost there. After the doctor was done, the technicians took me into recovery before I was released. My Dad and boyfriend weren't in sight. Where could they have gone? I was upset because someone needed to come soon to take a picture of the port before it was tossed into the trash. After about 10 minutes or so they arrived to recovery. I was so emotional by that time. They almost caused me to miss the opportunity to get my picture. That was near and dear to me. They came back with balloons and flowers but by that time I was already upset with them. I sent my boyfriend back to get the picture of the port. By the time he came back to me, it was time for me to get dressed and check out. I left excited all over again with a smile on my face. I took pictures that I shared with friends and family while headed back home. When I arrived, I rested up that evening and took in my day of surviving another surgery. It was another blessing along my survival journey.

Chapter 12:

An Ambassador and Advocate

*P*articipating in my first LRF walk in April of 2014 really lit a fire in me to stay involved with the organization. Over the years we forged a relationship that would catapult me to platforms I have never imagined. For example, prior to Cancer I dabbled in modeling (couple headshots) but nothing serious, lol. Fast forward to 2014, and as a part of my advocacy work, the Lymphoma Research Foundation invited me out to New York to shoot a very impactful campaign called "Erase Lymphoma". I was thrilled to get the invite. To have these types of opportunities to share my story on a platform that will give hope to others fighting like I once did, is a true testament of why God intended that I survived my fight.

My next experience with advocacy work came by way of venturing to California for my first Lymphoma Research

Foundation Educational Forum. I've never been to the west coast. I was happy about traveling to sunny California for the first time and attending a great event as a *Young Adult Ambassador*. I invited my boyfriend to come along with me. I figured we could explore the city of Los Angeles once my work was over. On top of that, he's so supportive so it would be a double win for me. Of course, when I told him without any hesitation, he said "Yes." We made such a great team. From there I jumped right into planning. I started looking into all types of things to do on my computer. I couldn't wait to leave. My boyfriend was just as thrilled as I was.

When we arrived in California, we grabbed our rental car and headed to the hotel where we would be staying. The educational forum with LRF was there too. We pulled up to the Marriott hotel and it was beautiful. The sun was shiny and the weather in California was great for the fall season. We went inside to check into the hotel and then proceeded to our room. It was a free day to settle in before the full day of events took place tomorrow morning so we decided to change out of our travel clothes and hit the city for some tourist action. As I sat on the edge of the bed while he showered, I took in this moment. It was a true blessing to be a part of this educational forum. The Lymphoma Research Foundation has given me great opportunities to be a part of the cancer communities as a survivor. I truly was thankful. We were both dressed and were ready to head out on the town for something to eat and sightseeing. We enjoyed our time out in the city. I got to see Hollywood Blvd, The Big Hollywood sign up on the hill that overlooks the entire city of Los Angeles and we grabbed some great food too. When we returned we changed into swimwear and sat out by the pool to relax a bit before dinner later this evening. I knew I didn't want to be up too late since the ambassador meeting started very early and would be a full day.

It was a beautiful Friday morning. I opened the curtains to let some sunlight shine into the room as I got dressed for my first ambassador meeting. I was so jolly as I wrapped my mind around meeting some amazing survivors and their loved ones as well. Also I was going to see the team from LRF again since my visit to New York. I got dressed and headed downstairs for breakfast. My boyfriend came along to support me. I could always count on him. He's so interested and invested in what makes me happy. You need that kind of support especially while trying to get through what I've been through. Breakfast was being served in the conference room where the meeting was being held. So when I arrived there were a few other ambassadors already sitting and eating or chatting with one another around the room. I introduced myself to them and greeted the staff members of LRF. My boyfriend and I grabbed a plate of food and sat to eat. Shortly after once everyone settled in, the meeting began.

The entire trip to the Lymphoma Research Foundation's Ed Forum was a success. I learned so much new and informative information pertaining to lymphoma disease. I got to meet other amazing survivors, current fighters, caregivers and the entire LRF staff. I was already looking forward to the next event.

To keep this ambassador/advocacy work going, over the summer, I decided to sign up for the Leukemia and Lymphoma Society *"Annual Light the Night Walk* "with my team, Dzire2Survive. The walk takes place all over the D.C., Maryland, and Virginia area throughout the month of October. It is for all cancer survivors, patients newly diagnosed, caregivers and their families. To raise Blood Cancer Awareness. My team and I worked together to raise money leading up to the walk day. We were successful to raise a great amount to help patients and their families financially. This was going to be my first walk with LLS. I was looking forward to it.

It was the day of the walk and my entire team showed up ready for a good time in the heart of D.C. There were so many attendees on the grounds of the monument. Music from local live bands. A fun area for kids. Food vendor trucks lined up on the street. It was an amazing sight to see. My team and I took lots and lots of cool pictures and had such a great time before the walk began. Once the sun set, it was time to walk from the monument down to the capital. The event's emcee acknowledged everyone for their outstanding support of survivors, current patients, those we have lost to this blood cancer disease and all caretakers. There were white, red, and yellow lanterns in the hands of attendees that can be seen all over the grounds. The countdown to begin walking started and once the emcee got to one, everyone cheered and took off.

The Light the Night walk was so much fun with my team and the other attendees. It was a very powerful celebration of one year being cancer free. I wanted to give back by participating in memorable walks for this amazing cause. I did just that alongside those close to me, and in support of my mission to give hope.

I started to receive invitations to share my story in several magazines and on online publications. It was a great feeling to be able to share within these outlets. I wanted to give the same hope I needed to their readers. That meant more to me than anything. Knowing that I could shine a light in my cancer communities all over the country and have an impact on so many lives. I decided to travel more for leisure. I felt it was the right thing to do since I knew personally now just how short life is. It was also a great way to spend quality time with my boyfriend. I was living my best life and I wanted nothing short of staying in complete remission.

Chapter 13:
The BIG 3-0

*M*y big 30th birthday was nearing in May of 2015. These last couple years of celebration including while I was battling cancer were relaxing. I was grateful to be alive and blessed to see another year. This year was big so I wanted to plan something fun and phenomenal. I put together a big dinner party at a hot restaurant and lounge in D.C. with all of my loved ones. I also planned a fabulous vacation to beautiful Jamaica. The plans were set and I am ready to celebrate. I got a beautiful custom red dress made that would stop traffic for my dinner party and all. It was nothing like being able to look back at where I started a short time ago to where I was currently in my life. This was truly a milestone to celebrate. One of my girlfriends and I share the same birthday so we agreed to have our dinner party together.

We have been friends since high school and having the same birthday was like being birth twins.

It was the day of my dinner party and I was ready to rock and roll. I had all types of things to do to prepare. Like get my hair, nails, and makeup done. I knew I would be running around doing these things but I wasn't worried one bit. I scheduled my appointments accordingly. It seemed like the night came quickly. I was ready to get dressed and head out with my man by my side. When I came down the stairs, he told me how beautiful I looked. He took pictures of me and then we headed out to the dinner. When we arrived, everyone else attending was arriving as well. They all looked so amazing in their evening attire. We greeted each other and took pictures as the DJ was blazing the hottest hits in the background. Once we sat at the dining table that had 20 guests, we began to order our food and cocktails. Everyone was having a good time. We ate, laughed and danced the evening away. The party was lots of fun. It was very late when we left the restaurant and my boyfriend and I had an early morning flight to Jamaica in just a few short hours. When we got back to the house, I finished up my packing. Then I laid down for a little before it was time to head for the airport.

It was vacation time. I was excited but a little tired from the night before. I was ready to enjoy a week away on the beach with lots of fun in the sun. We got up and headed to the airport for our flights. It was early morning so when we arrived, there weren't many travelers. That meant not a long wait to check in or to get through the security. The process was short and sweet. Jamaica, here we come!! When I arrived and checked in I was ready to let my hair down. We were staying at a beautiful all-inclusive adult's only resort in Ochos Rios, Jamaica. The staff were really pleasant, and the oceanfront was breathtaking. I couldn't ask for a better way to celebrate my 30th birthday. We got our tropical drinks and set out by the poolside. Tomorrow we had a full day of excursions planned. I couldn't wait to enjoy myself.

I loved my stay in Jamaica. We did some fun tourist excursions, ate lots of great Caribbean foods, danced to the Caribbean beats and overall enjoyed being with one another.

Chapter 14:

Loading...

I was a woman evolving every step of the way. I was happy with my progress at this time in my life. I attended women empowerment events to better myself as a woman and as a person. I also wanted to find new outlets outside of cancer communities to network with. I wanted to work with others that were doing great things in the community. Business owners, speakers, spiritually connected individuals and just across the board well rounded like-minded people with similar goals. All of which could help me continue to grow. I knew in this moment it was time for me to find platforms to share my story. I really wanted to uplift other cancer fighters and those with their own set of adversities. I knew it was time for me to do more in my community. So in order to grow and be a better me, I had to attend events and get in the know by networking.

I was beginning to feel like I was being affected by what I thought I'd overcome with cancer. I didn't know what this feeling was. I remember having anxiety but this feeling was somewhat different. I would cry silently to myself. I would feel sad. I would feel like I was still fighting for my life and the feeling was uneasy to me. Sometimes I didn't even want to be bothered with my boyfriend. Although he was able to grasp a lot of what went on in my day to day life, I was still battling a lot on the inside. He wanted me to feel free to express myself even more. But there were some issues that I still didn't even have control over yet. That caused friction in our relationship. He didn't know what was going on with me. It was hard to explain. I just wanted to deal with these feelings alone and in my own way. No doctor, no sharing with anyone else, not even him. Just kept it all to myself.

It was June 2015. I was invited by a fellow cancer survivor and model to participate in an awareness fashion event "Alive Again". This would be my first time hitting a runway. Getting made over with beautiful makeup and some unique fashion pieces was a great first time experience. I was nervous because I had never been in the spotlight like this before. I invited my Mom and my boyfriend to come out and support me. It being my first time doing a fashion show, I showed out on the runway like I was a vet. My Mom and boyfriend were cheering me on as I walked by in my stylish designs by some dope clothing designers. I thought to myself, "Maybe I can do this more often," I always wanted to be a model. I was always very curvy with a few extra pounds so I didn't think I would be accepted into the fashion world as one. After that event I decided to get into modeling. I did the research and started to network with photographers and other models to get into the industry. I wanted to get my feet wet to see what modeling was all about.

While I was taking on this new found direction into modeling, I was also working on some other projects through my movement Dzire2Survive. I wanted to create a journal line for newly diagnosed patients and survivors as a space to write and or doodle in throughout their personal journeys. I did some digging and found an incredible lady with a small business through etsy.com. She helped me to create the design look I needed. The designing process was great. We discussed my vision for my journals and every step of the way she helped me bring it to life. I was thrilled to start getting these journals out into the hands of others. I was beginning to get creative in what I wanted to see for my brand. I wanted to help others affected by cancer. I wanted to give them a safe space to talk about what they've been through. I want to be a face and voice for those in need of hope, and courage to fight cancer back and win.

After my journals were custom handmade, I signed up and attended events. This allowed me to set up my table to sell my journals and lanyards. Each one came with inspirational and encouraging wording on them. It was also my way of connecting all while finding my lane in the business communities. I wanted nothing more than to continue to learn as a movement creator and cancer advocate.

Chapter 15:

My Life Flashes Again

I was invited to audition for some fashion events. To my surprise, I was chosen to participate as a model. I was so happy. I didn't think I would be chosen especially as a curvy girl. It was the start of my modeling career. I did an event for cancer awareness at Lord and Taylor. I did a few photoshoots to begin building my portfolio. I was having fun with the start of my new modeling career. I was still finding time to travel and focus on my Dzire2Survive movement as well.

It was the start of my work day. Up at the crack of dawn like any other morning at 4am and ready to get moving into the office. I got into my work uniform and headed out the door. It was 5 am and it seemed like so many people were on the road.

As I was driving on highway 95 north, after about 10 minutes or so, a vehicle in front of me slammed on their brakes. It caused me to slam onto mine and then out of nowhere another vehicle slammed into the back of my car. It caused my car to fishtail outward across four lanes.

The impact was so intense that my entire body lifted out of my driver seat. It tossed me over causing my neck to hit the edge of my passenger seat. I lost complete control of the steering wheel until my car came to a complete stop in the middle of the highway. I saw my life flash before my eyes, again. I thought that the other vehicles and tractor trailers traveling northbound towards me were going to crash into me as well. I sat sideways in the middle of the highway shaking uncontrollably. I couldn't move because of the impact. My adrenaline was on full throttle. I was looking over to the opposite side of the highway where the other car was. I saw the driver of the car that hit me jumping up and down tossing his hand in the air upset. After a few moments an ambulance arrived at the scene. The paramedic opened my driver side door and asked if I was able to move. I said, "No". He then went to get a back board and neck brace to remove me from the car to put me into the ambulance. This would allow them to take me to the nearest hospital. I was still panicking from the accident. I had never been in a collision like this before. All I could think about while lying inside the back of the ambulance was how grateful I was that it wasn't worse. Before the ambulance left the scene, an officer came in to get my driver's license to write a report. Then he stated that he would return it to me at the hospital. I asked the EMT which hospital they were taking me to because I did not want to go to Prince George's Hospital. (Sidebar: This hospital does not have the best reputation in the area where I live. I've heard some unpleasant things about it, and I can deal with cancer and a car accident, but I COULD NOT deal with having to be treated at that place). To my dismay, the EMT said exactly where I didn't want to go, PG hospital. He replied that the other hospitals were not accepting any ambulance emergencies. I was mortified but what could I do?

We arrived at Prince General Hospital's E.R. entrance a short time later. A nurse came out from behind the counter to meet us. As I was lying there, I overheard the paramedic. He said that they were actually headed to another emergency call when they saw my car stopped in the middle of the highway. All I could think was how lucky I was. I was taken back to a room to have my vitals checked and observation of my injuries from the accident. I was in some pain, but I knew it would be 10x worse tomorrow. I was not looking forward to it. I called my work because I knew they were wondering why I hadn't arrived for my shift yet. I told them what just happened to me. Then I called my boyfriend. He was up getting ready for work. He sounded so scared over the phone but I assured him that my injuries were minor. He was on his way up to the hospital once he called in to work. After I got off the phone with him, I called my family and told them. My Mom was on her way (my Dad was out of town, so she was coming alone).

As I was sitting in the hospital bed I was wondering if my car was totaled and how long would it be before I got back to work. I knew I would be in some physical pain that would keep me home for a bit. The E.R. doctor came in to speak with me. He told me that I had some minor injuries to my neck and prescribed meds to pick up for the pain. A few seconds later, the officer from earlier walked in with my driver's license and the tow yard information to where my car was located. I was given my discharge documents. Then the officer and doctor walked out. I waited in the room until my Mom and boyfriend arrived to pick me up.

It was perfect timing because they both came at the same time. We left and headed to the pharmacy to pick my meds up so that I could go home to relax. The next day as expected, I was in so much pain. It felt like a mac truck hit me and I could barely move. I got up to have breakfast and to take some medication to relieve some of the pain. Next, I reached out to my car insurance company to see if my car would be totaled. I needed to know my next steps. I was on the phone for about 30 minutes or so with a representative. She gave me information on getting a rental car. She also confirmed that my car was totaled from the accident. I sensed that would be the case. My car was older and for the most part getting it fixed would be expensive.

I know things happen for a reason but this took the cake. For a few weeks now I would see the Chevy Malibu commercial and say to myself, "I want that car." Then this accident happens where my car gets destroyed. Go figure this would be the outcome. I was happy but also not pleased. Now I have to purchase a new car, and have a car note after not having one for a few years now. But hey, guess who was headed to the dealership to get the car they had been wanting for a couple weeks now? See how God works?! I was lucky on that highway. It could have been a tragedy if it had gone another way.

Chapter 16:

Getting Back on Track

It's beautiful springtime of 2016 (my favorite season) and I was continuing with my advocacy and outreach work. I auditioned a few months prior for my first curvy fashion event "District of Curves" and was selected to be a part of the show. The experience was phenomenal. So many beautiful curvy women hit the runway and slayed the curvy and plus fashion styles like queens. I got to meet and network with some awesome individuals at the show. I was ecstatic about the experience and looking forward to the next year to audition again.

Soon thereafter I would learn that I would be honored at the "Church Girls Rock" awards as a Cancer Survivor and Community Advocate. This award means so much to me because of the adversities I had overcome and still pushing through each day as a survivor of cancer. When I got the call to be recognized I couldn't compose myself. I was happier than a kid in a candy store. My family, one of my good girlfriends and my boyfriend were all so happy for me. They purchased their tickets to attend and I couldn't be more blessed to have them support this honor. I had to find the perfect dress for this day. I had to also prepare a few words to share once I went up to receive my award. I was a nervous mess thinking about speaking in front of an auditorium full of people, but I was ready to share my story with everyone.

It was awards day and I was ready to get into my beautiful gown. I couldn't wait to have my hair and makeup done for another special moment in my life. After getting glammed for this big day, my boyfriend and I headed out to the venue. He told me how beautiful I looked, as he always did. I must say, we looked good as a unit going to this event. We made it to the venue where the event was being held. They had a red carpet once you walked in so that the honorees and their families could take pictures before the program began. After taking a few photos, we walked inside the auditorium and sat down in our assigned seats. A short time later, we listened to the emcee speak about the "Church Girls Rock" program. Then she started to read the bios and introduce the honorees of the evening. I waited nervously for my bio to be read. When it was my turn to go up, the emcee read mine. The slideshow of pictures on the big screen in the background was showing images of myself, and some with my family. Once she was done reading my bio about me, she called my name. I was escorted by my boyfriend up on stage. I walked up to receive my award as the entire audience applauded me. I gave my speech and it felt good hearing myself share tough moments of my life with others. The event was great and I couldn't be more proud to be honored.

Fast forward to October 2016 and it was time for the Leukemia and Lymphoma Society's annual "Light the Night" walk again. I wanted to be a part of this walk every year. I got my team together again for another great walk. This year was particularly special though because in the year prior my Aunt had been diagnosed with non-Hodgkin's Lymphoma was also a survivor. She overcame her second battle against the disease over the summer, so I wanted to dedicate this walk to her. Our entire family and friends came together on this day to walk in her honor, and we had a blast again like before. The event is always lots of fun for the entire family to enjoy. There I was with another cancer awareness walk under my belt, yet so much more to do to help continue to raise awareness in my community.

Chapter 17:

"The Atmosphere Was Shifting"

I was beginning to see a shift in my life. I never thought I would be faced with these types of adversities. It was starting to affect my daily thoughts and day to day activities. I was often having depression and anxiety. I didn't have a good feeling about things. There are many days I find myself feeling off and thinking a lot about what transpired over the past 3 years. I was beginning to also see my features changing. At first I didn't know why, but after some research I found that I had some hyper-pigmentation (discoloration, dark circles around my eyes and some other small blemishes). I became very self-conscious with how I started to see myself in the mirror. It made me sad and scared to walk out the house without some type of makeup to cover my blemishes. It may not be a big deal to some but I felt like I was unattractive.

I began to see the changes. To face depression and now this, it was a lot for me personally.

I started to search to find ways to cope without having to see a therapist about what I was experiencing. I didn't want to share my battle with anyone so I just found different avenues to get through it on my own. What seems to help is my cancer awareness movement and modeling career. Modeling is my safe haven. It keeps me grounded. I also looked more into what types of makeup brands I could purchase to cover the changes with my face. I didn't think I needed to over stress the situation but I wanted to keep it under control overall.

I continued to work on my Dzire2Survive brand and wanted to do something different for kids affected by the cancer disease. Now that the Christmas season was approaching, I wanted to give to children diagnosed with cancer. I contacted my Auntie who works as a nurse at a Children's Hospital to see if she'll be able to connect me with a family in need. She was happy to help me with my project. My friends and family donated toys and monetary gifts to help me. It turned out amazing. I made arrangements with the child's family to bring all of the gifts over for the little fighter. A few days later, I arrived at the family house and I got to meet the tough cookie. He was shy at first. He became very excited once he saw all of his gifts. The family was so happy and very thankful that I could help at this time. I was more than happy to be a blessing in their lives at this tough time.

Going into 2017 I was optimistic and continued my education and outreach efforts, but out of nowhere, in the Spring of 2017 tragedy struck my entire family. I never imagined I would ever lose someone so close to me at such a young age, but my older cousin passed away from an apparent overdose. It was Sunday morning. I went over to my parent's house to visit for a bit. My Mom went upstairs to grab something for me. Then when she came back downstairs she was crying hysterically saying something happened to my cousin. She was deceased. She went on to say that my Dad just got a call from my Aunt (my Dad's sister). She was screaming and crying. She found my cousin in her apartment unresponsive after not hearing from her for a few days. I became instantly frozen as I was trying to take in what my mom was saying to me. My boyfriend was sitting in the living room. He jumped up to come see what was going on. I started to cry and tried calling my Aunt myself to see if this was all true. When she answered she was screaming and crying so I hung up. I asked my boyfriend to take me over to my cousin's place. My family was right behind us.

We left the house quickly to go over to her home where my Aunt found her alongside her son. I was so devastated and couldn't believe what was happening. This was my big cousin and nothing has ever happened like this in our family before. It was very painful for all of us. When we got there other family members were already outside her apartment. My Aunt and the police officers were still inside. More relatives received the news and were pulling up to the scene. After standing outside for what seemed like an eternity, the coroner arrived. They took out the stretcher from the back with a black body bag. We all lost it and started to really break down into tears. We knew they were about to get my cousin's body ready to bring her out.

Once they went inside the apartment for about 20 minutes or so, we saw the door open. They were coming out with my cousin's body. Her mom was crying as she was being held up by her son. I was so heartbroken seeing her body brought out. This sudden tragedy was hard for me for several days after. I took a day or two off from work. I cried so much everyday thinking about my cousin and her sudden death. It wasn't easy but over time, each day I became a little better than the last. This gave me perspective; life can be taken in an instant, and after everything I had endured to that point, at times questioning my own mortality, I made my mind up that for every day I was granted I would LIVE to the best of my abilities.

Chapter 18:

The Evolving Woman

I was approaching my 5-year survival anniversary. This date meant so much to me because the survival rate was small for the type of cancer I was diagnosed with. I was blessed to see five years of survival. I decided to plan a nice celebration with close friends and family. I planned a nice private dinner at Ruth Chris. I invited those that continuously supported my journey from the very beginning. The survival dinner went over well. We indulged in much laugher, great conversations and most importantly, a celebration of life.

More and more I was growing. Not just as a woman but as a person overall. I faced some trials along the way. My battle against depression, anxiety and beauty were some challenges that persisted. I was working to tackle these insecurities each day and had come so far, but still had work to do. In dealing with some of those challenges, I lost some relationships. One of which included the relationship with my then fiancé. Trying to fight my own personal battles and keep a strong foundation became too much. I decided that it was best we parted ways. I wanted to work on me and become a better person for me first.

I found ways to balance so that I could avoid being overwhelmed. I auditioned for DC Fashion Week for the first time and was selected to walk for several designers in the show. The show was a great experience. This opportunity let me know that I was moving up in the modeling world. From New York Fashion Week to DSW Fashion Shoe store's first fashion show as part of a campaign alongside the women empowerment company, Create & Cultivate. I was blessed to be able to continue to share my story on different platforms. Like being invited to speak on the mainstage at the Lymphoma Research Foundation's Educational Forum in Chicago. That was a very special accomplishment in my career as a speaker and survivor. I was a proud woman evolving in such phenomenal ways.

Perseverance

I didn't quite think that I would face other difficulties such as depression and anxiety following my survival with cancer. But with depression led to issues in my relationships. With anxiety led to me often worrying about my future and if the cancer would come back. Then another life altering challenge came knocking on my life's door, Uterine Fibroids. After months of tremendous pain and a heavy menstrual cycle, I finally decided to see my OBGYN for some answers as to why I was all of a sudden having these issues. After my consultation with her and a referral to have an ultrasound done, I left the doctor's office. Shortly after, I called the radiology center to schedule my appointment. My appointment was made for the following week. I couldn't take any more of this pain I was experiencing in the pit of my stomach each month like clockwork.

It was the day for my ultrasound. I was concerned and didn't know what to expect. Not too long after checking in, I was escorted to an examined room to prepare for my ultrasound. The technician rubbed warm gel over my belly and proceeded to slowly roll a wand across my belly. Moments later after getting a few images, she inserted the wand into my happy place as well which threw me completely off. It was a weird experience. The technician called for some assistance and someone else came into the dark room to help her. The technician that came into the room slipped up by asking if I was there for my "Fibroids?" I was devastated by what she asked. I didn't think that would be the outcome. She quickly became silent and proceeded taking images while the hard object was still inserted inside of me.

A little while later they were done. I wiped off and got dressed to leave. Both technicians were standing outside of the room waiting. They told me that I should hear from my doctor's office in a few days and showed me the way out. When I left, all I could think about was what the technician said to me. "Fibroids...fibroids?!" This explains my painful menstrual each month. Needless to say, a few days later that was the case. I had two fibroids and a small cyst surrounding my uterus. My OBGYN doctor assured me that I would be ok and that many women like me live with them. She told me the things I could do to keep them from becoming enlarged and ways to cope each month with my cycles.

I truly felt like I was being attacked with different challenges. They began taking over my mental space and sometimes my day to day activities. That's a whole other story I'll share with you soon... but just know that like with Cancer, this is a fight that I'm willing to go 12-rounds for if I have to.

Conclusion

*P*resently, I am at a good point in my life. I have grown so much and evolved tremendously as a woman. From surviving stage 4 cancer, to finding my love for modeling and making it a career, to magazine features and my first magazine cover in January 2020 sharing my amazing life changing story, building my cancer advocacy movement, Dzire2Survive and so much more. I have had my share of ups and downs, but I stayed faithful to His word. I kept going through it all. My struggles are a part of my journey that has helped me to understand that I am human. It's what keeps me grounded and finding positive outlets to keep me evolving each and every day. I have started a movement called "Feel Beautiful Look Beautiful". It encourages young girls and women affected by cancer to see that they are beautiful and bold in every way. It will give them HOPE and the COURAGE to see their beauty throughout their cancer journey, as well as life after cancer. I plan to make a difference and be the change I want to see in others. While it is not yet written (literally in this book or figuratively) I have a great plan for my next chapter and I know fully that with God, anything is possible!

A Road To Recovery

Etiquette 101: How To Support Someone Living With Cancer

I am often asked many questions by people that have family members newly diagnosed with cancer or just typical cancer related questions whenever I share with someone that I am a cancer survivor. Questions like, "How was the journey for you?" "Did you lose your hair?" "Did you lose weight?" "Were you often sick and fatigue?" For someone that's newly diagnosed, you can't even begin to explain what you need at that time. You don't really know yourself during that time, but you do know that you want to survive your battle against this disease called Cancer.

Emotional support is paramount for a cancer patient. That's the part that can be hard for most individuals, especially when it's your close relatives learning about your diagnosis for the very first time as well. The experience is in fact new for everyone and can be very difficult (as you could imagine). Despite this, I find it normal for relatives and/or friends of newly diagnosed cancer patients to inquire about what's happening and to seek information. I think that providing a resource created by someone like myself that has experienced the cancer journey personally would be hugely helpful. As a survivor, I enjoy answering these often-asked questions as I feel it is very informative and helpful for many.

Many cancer survivors share similar stories of awkward encounters and upsetting comments made by well-meaning individuals. Their observations help many define "cancer etiquette," or rules of conduct for communicating with the cancer community. Many individuals experience cancer differently, one approach does not necessarily work for everyone. This information serves as a starting point for talking to someone with cancer. There is no single right way but keep going until you finally get it. Get It?

As such, I'm providing a list that I think could be helpful for advocates (friends and family) of cancer patients called: "Support Etiquette 101". I've compiled these tips on the next couple of pages.

"Support Etiquette 101: Helpful Tips for Cancer Advocates"

Good Etiquette 101-1. Don't ignore them. Some people disappear when someone they know gets cancer. The worst thing you can do is avoid the person because you don't know how to handle it. Cancer can be lonely and isolating as it is. Tell them:

"I'm here for you, " or "I love you, and we'll get through this together."

It's even okay to say: "I don't know what to say" OR send a note that says, "I'm thinking of you." Just stay connected.

Good Etiquette 101-2. Think before you speak. Your words and actions can be powerful. One comment can instantly undo someone's positive mood. Don't be overly grave and mournful. Avoid clichés, like "hero" and "battle." If the person gets worse, does it mean they didn't fight hard enough? Try to imagine if you were in your friend's shoes. What you would want someone to say to you?

Good Etiquette 101-3. Follow their lead. Let the person with cancer set the tone about what he or she wants to talk about. It doesn't always have to be about cancer. Chances are your friend wants to feel as normal as possible. Tell him or her about something funny that happened. Allow your friend to talk about cancer if he or she wants. And save the pity eyes and voice.

Good Etiquette 101-4. Keep it about your friend, not you. Don't lose your focus. Avoid talking about your headache, backache, etc. This isn't about you. And as bad as you feel, he or she feels worse and may not be interested in hearing about how hard this has been on your life. Don't put him or her in the position of having to comfort you. Only ask questions if you truly want to hear the response.

Good Etiquette 101-5. Just listen. Sometimes just being there to listen—really listen— is the best thing you can do. Let the person with cancer talk without interrupting. You don't always have to have all the answers, just a sympathetic ear. He or she may not want to talk at all, and would rather sit quietly. It's okay to sit in silence.

Good Etiquette 101-6. Don't minimize their experience. Try not to say, "Don't worry, you'll be fine." You don't know that. Instead say, "I'm really sorry, " or "I hope it will be okay." And don't refer to his or her cancer as "the good cancer." These statements downplay what he or she is going through. Leave the door to communication open so they can talk about fears and concerns.

Good Etiquette 101-7. Don't be intrusive. Don't ask those with cancer questions about their numbers or tumor markers. If they want to talk about their blood results, they will. Give them the freedom to offer this information or not. Also, don't ask personal questions that you wouldn't have asked before, especially when it comes to subjects like sex and religion.

Good Etiquette 101-8. Don't preach to them. Don't try to tell the person with cancer what to think, feel or how to act. You don't know what they're going through, so don't act like you do. Instead of saying "I know how you feel, " try saying "I care about you and want to help." Don't suggest alternative forms of treatment, a healthier lifestyle, etc. And don't tell them to "stay positive, " it will only cause frustration and guilt.

Good Etiquette 101-9. Refrain from physical assessments. Refrain from comments about how those with cancer look, particularly if it's negative. They don't need their weight loss or hair loss pointed out to them. And if they just started treatment, don't ask them about potential side effects. If you say anything at all, tell them they look stronger or more beautiful, but mean what you say.

Good Etiquette 101-10. Avoid comparisons. Everyone does cancer his or her own way. Don't bring up the private medical problems of other people you know. And don't talk about your friend with cancer who is running marathons or never missed a day of work. Avoid talking about the odds or making assumptions about prognosis. Just allow your friend to be who they are.

Good Etiquette 101-11. Show them you care. Show those with cancer that they're still needed and loved. Give them a hug. Surprise them with a smoothie, books, magazines or music. Offer to help, such as cooking, laundry, babysitting or running errands. Be specific by asking, "What day can I bring you dinner?" And, offer to help only if you intend to follow through with it and won't expect something in return.

Good Etiquette 101-12. Share encouraging stories. Offer encouragement through success stories of long-term cancer survivors. Avoid saying, "They had the same thing as you." No two cancers are the same. And never tell stories with unhappy endings. If you know someone with the same type of cancer, offer to connect the two of them.

(Source: Cancer Treatment Center of America, Cancer Etiquette, www.cancercenters.com)

I *highly recommend* the websites of the **Lymphoma Research Foundation** at http://www.lymphoma.org ; **The Leukemia and Lymphoma Society** at http://www.lls.org and **The American Cancer Society** at http://www.cancer.org

Acknowledgements

I Survived was a lesson of courage, resilience, and faith. I began writing down every obstacle I endured in my last days of treatments in September of 2013. I didn't want to forget each moment that made me the survivor and woman I am today. It took me 7 years to get the courage to put my experience with cancer into a book and out into the universe but I must say, I am very happy that I decided to do so. I Survived shows true perseverance and gives you the true definition of a fighter. I wrote every word on each page with hopes that it inspires every reader in such a way that gives you the courage to be resilient.

To my family and friends, thank you for being a part of my survival journey from the very beginning and today, as I continue to embark this incredible path that continues to lead me into the direction I want to be.

To my Mom and Dad, thank you for everything you've taught me as a young girl that makes me the woman that I am today. Fearless!! Thank you for being by my side along my cancer journey the entire way (doctor's appointments, chemotherapy treatments, etc.) and all of my needs that you continue to help me through in life.

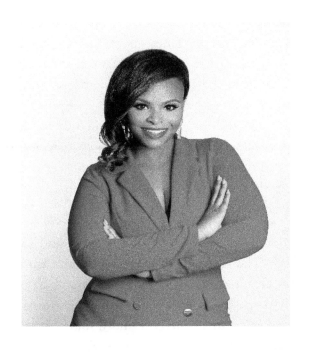

About the Author

Erica Campbell was born and raised in Washington, D.C. to her parents Eric Campbell and Vanessa Holloway. Erica is the second oldest of five siblings. Erica is an Aunt of five nieces and nephews who she truly loves.

Through her unwavering faith and trust in God as well as exuding a positive attitude, Erica knew she could get through it all. Since overcoming her battle with cancer, she has set a new path in life. In 2014, Erica founded "Dzire2Survive": a cancer support and advocacy movement that helps improve the quality of life of patients and their families touched by the lymphoma disease, by providing education and up to date information. Erica wants to inspire patients with peer to peer comfort and hope to help them continue to fight and overcome their battle with blood cancers.

Erica is an ambassador with "The Leukemia and Lymphoma Society" and "The Lymphoma Research Foundation" where her story is featured on their Adolescent and Young Adult stories of hope page (https://www.lymphoma.org). Erica has been featured as a cancer survivor and fashion cover model in magazines and digital feature outlets sharing her life changing story such as Sheen Magazine, Plus Model Magazine, HelloBeautiful, Luxe Magazine, Houston Style Magazine, Healthline, Cancer Today Magazine, CURE Magazine, and with a host of other special features including the Lymphoma Research Foundation's Lymphoma Awareness Campaign videos (Erase Lymphoma, Impacting Lives-Youtube).

In April 2014 and 2015 and Oct 2014-2019, Erica raised funds to help financially assist newly diagnosed patients and their families with her team "Dzire2Survive" as they impacted so many lives at the Light the Night Walk with the Leukemia and Lymphoma Society and the Lymphoma 5k Walk with the Lymphoma Research Foundation.

Today, Erica continues her journey as Inspirational Speaker, Patient Advocate, Self-Love Influencer and Model. Erica has shared her survival story on many inspirational platforms as well as her rising modeling career as she continues to grow in both runway and editorial fashion.

In Erica's spare time she loves to travel to beautiful destinations and most of all spending time with her family and close friends. Erica loves the Lord and through Him, she enjoys helping others affected by cancer and other life adversities by sharing her empowering story.

Erica's motto that she loves to share with other fighters and survivors is,

"Never give up your fight and continue to survive with your beautiful smile."

Always have a Dzire2Survive.

Author's Note

I am so thankful that you chose my book, "I Survived" to read. It's very humbling.

I'd like to ask of you a BIG favor…

I am really working hard to get some amazing reviews, you know, to keep pushing the boundaries!

Can you help me do that?

If you like the book… and if you would be willing to spare just two or three minutes…would you be willing to share your review of the book on the outlet in which you purchased (Amazon, Barnes & Nobles) (if you haven't done so already)?

You can also send your thoughts directly to me via email at info@ericasurvived.com

If you would, it would mean the absolute world to me!

This helps me get my book into as many hands as possible, helping others to Never Give Up and Keep Surviving!

I really appreciate all your support, you guys rock.

CPSIA information can be obtained
at www.ICGtesting.com
Printed in the USA
LVHW020901020421
683299LV00004B/226